Caring for a cat with lower urinary tract disease

by Dr Sarah Caney and Professor Danièlle Gunn-Moore

Published by Vet Professionals 2014

Copyright © Vet Professionals 2014

www.vetprofessionals.com

ISBN 978-1-908583-06-2

About Cat Professional

Cat Professional is a subdivision of Vet Professionals Ltd. Cat Professional was founded in 2007 by Dr Sarah Caney with the aims of providing cat owners and veterinary professionals with the highest quality information, advice, training and consultancy services.

Publications

Cat Professional is a leading provider of high quality publications on caring for cats with a variety of medical conditions. Written by international experts in their field, each book is written to be understood by cat owners and veterinary professionals. The books are available to buy through the website www.vetprofessionals.com as eBooks where they can be downloaded and read instantly. Alternatively they can be purchased as a softback via the website and good bookstores.

'Caring for a cat with lower urinary tract disease' was first published in January 2009. This updated third edition was published in March 2014. Other books in the Cat Professional series include:

- 'Caring for a cat with chronic kidney disease' by Dr Sarah Caney
- 'Caring for a blind cat' by Natasha Mitchell
- 'Caring for a cat with hyperthyroidism' by Dr Sarah Caney
- 'Caring for an overweight cat' by Andrea Harvey and Samantha Taylor

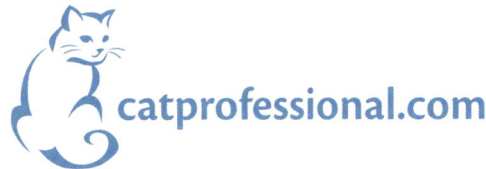

A variety of free-to-download articles also feature on the Vet Professionals website.

Advice, Training and Consultancy

Cat Professional is dedicated to improving the standards of cat care and in this capacity is a provider of Continuing Professional Development to veterinary surgeons, veterinary nurses and other professionals working with cats around the world.

Cat Professional also works closely with leading providers of cat products and foods providing training programmes, assisting with product literature and advising on product design and marketing.

Specialist feline medicine advice is available to veterinary professionals and cat owners world-wide. Details are available on the website.

About the authors

Sarah Caney (pictured right) is an internationally recognised veterinary specialist in feline medicine who has worked as a feline-only vet since 1994. She trained as a specialist at the University of Bristol, England and is one of only fourteen recognised specialists in feline medicine working within the UK. Sarah has written many articles for veterinarians and cat owners and works very closely with the cat charity, International Cat Care, (www.icatcare.org). Sarah has written two other books published by Cat Professional – 'Caring for a cat with chronic kidney disease' and 'Caring for a cat with hyperthyroidism'. As a clinician she enjoys seeing a mixture of first opinion and referral feline patients. She has been invited to lecture on feline medicine at veterinary conferences all over the world. Sarah lives in Scotland and has a handsome moggy called Sooty (pictured below right).

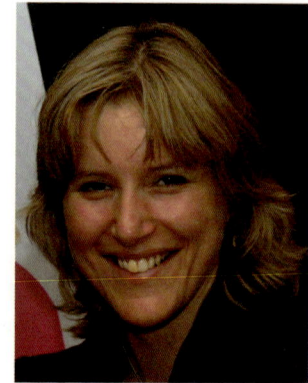

Danièlle Gunn-Moore is an internationally recognised veterinary specialist in feline medicine who graduated with Distinction from the R(D)SVS, University of Edinburgh, in 1991. For the last fourteen years she has been based at the University of Edinburgh where she set up the Feline Clinic and is now a Professor of Feline Medicine. Danièlle is an internationally recognised expert in her area, lectures extensively and her work has been published widely. In 2009, she was awarded the BSAVA Woodrow Award for outstanding contribution in the field of small animal veterinary medicine; in 2011, she was awarded the International Society for Feline Medicine/Hill's award for outstanding contributions to Feline Medicine. She shares her home with her husband Frank and two beautiful cats; an elderly Bengal girl called Teaninich and a Maine Coon boy called Mortlach (both named after Scottish single malt whiskies). Danièlle is pictured (right) with Mortlach.

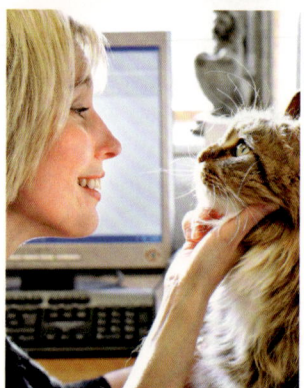

About this book

This book has been written as both a printed book and an interactive electronic book.

Words in blue are contained in the glossary section at the end of the book.

Dedications and acknowledgements

Thanks go to Sarah Heath of Behaviour Referrals (Chester, UK) for her invaluable help with the behavioural information included in this book.

The pictures included in this book are the copyright of the authors with two exceptions. The picture of Danièlle (this page and back cover) is included with kind permission of the University of Edinburgh; Josh (pictured page 50) is included with permission of his owner.

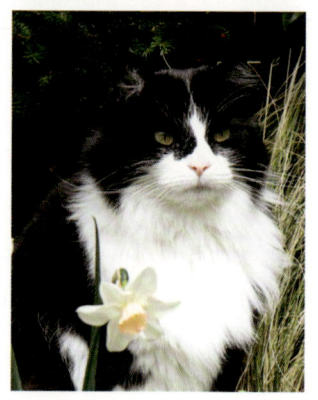

CONTENTS

FOREWORD 6

INTRODUCTION 7

SECTION 1 | the emotional side of things 8
Receiving bad news: coping with the emotional side of receiving a diagnosis of lower urinary tract disease in your cat 8

SECTION 2 | explaining the science of lower urinary tract disease 12
What is feline lower urinary tract disease (FLUTD)? 12
What is the urinary tract? 12
What causes FLUTD? 12
What is periuria? 20
What causes urethral obstruction? 22
Can FLUTD be prevented? 23
How can I tell if my cat is stressed? 23
What are the signs of FLUTD? 24
How is FLUTD diagnosed? 24
What other tests are helpful in cats with FLUTD? 31
How is FLUTD treated? 32
What surgical treatment options are there? 47
What is the prognosis (long-term outlook) for cats with FLUTD? 48

SECTION 3 | case illustration 49
Josh: a cat whose FLUTD is successfully managed by his owner 49

SECTION 4 | discussing your cat with your vet 51

SECTION 5 | further information 52
Knowing when to say 'goodbye' 52
How to cope with losing your cat 54

Useful websites and further reference sources 56

Glossary of terms used by vets 57

Converting SI units to Conventional units and vice versa 63

FOREWORD

Feline lower urinary tract disease (FLUTD) affects up to 10% of pet cats and is typically characterised by episodes of cystitis with affected cats passing small amounts of bloody urine, often showing pain and difficulty when doing so. FLUTD can be caused by many conditions including bladder stones and infections. In these cases, successful treatment depends on identifying and treating the cause of the problem. However, the majority of affected cats suffer from idiopathic FLUTD (also known as FIC – feline idiopathic cystitis) – in other words FLUTD without an identifiable underlying cause. Unlike many other medical conditions, there is no single effective treatment for FIC cases and certainly no 'magic pill' that can cure their illness. Instead, successful management depends upon a long-term commitment and team approach between owner, veterinarian and cat. Research studies have shown that it is possible to greatly reduce the frequency and severity of episodes of FIC for the vast majority of affected cats through:

- Identifying and addressing any potential sources of stress to the affected cat. Common examples include tension between the affected cat and others in the household/neighbourhood. A successful strategy in this example might be to ensure that there are sufficient litter boxes to enable unrestricted access without the concern that a 'bullying' cat might be able to prevent a vulnerable FIC cat from accessing the litter box

- Pursuing tactics that help the cat to produce more dilute urine. These include strategies to encourage the cat to drink more (such as use of water fountains and flavoured water) and use of specially designed prescription diets which also encourage drinking

- Additional treatments may be needed in some FIC cats and include painkillers and medication to treat urethral spasm

Whilst FIC is not an easy problem to resolve, attention to all of the above is usually successful in at least reducing the frequency and severity of episodes. In around three quarters of cases of FIC, the above treatment will result in a 'cure'.

Recent innovations which have greatly improved treatment success include the development of specially formulated veterinary prescription diets which are able to treat FLUTD in many ways. Use of these diets can dissolve some bladder stones (avoiding the necessity for surgery) and help prevent new bladder stones from forming. Both dry and canned formulations of some of these diets can be extremely effective in helping cats to produce less concentrated urine.

Dr Sarah Caney and Professor Danièlle Gunn-Moore

INTRODUCTION

Overall, lower urinary tract disease is thought to affect at least 1% of patients registered to a UK, US or European veterinary practice at any one time. Some studies have indicated that figures for indoor cats are as high as 10%. Incidence figures are not available for other countries but it is likely that a similar rate of disease is seen. It is a cause of considerable distress to affected cats and their owners.

This guide has been written to provide cat owners with the information they need to understand this complex condition and provide the best care for their cat. The authors regularly lecture on this subject and the contents of this book reflect what they teach to veterinary students, veterinary nurses, technicians and qualified veterinary surgeons around the world.

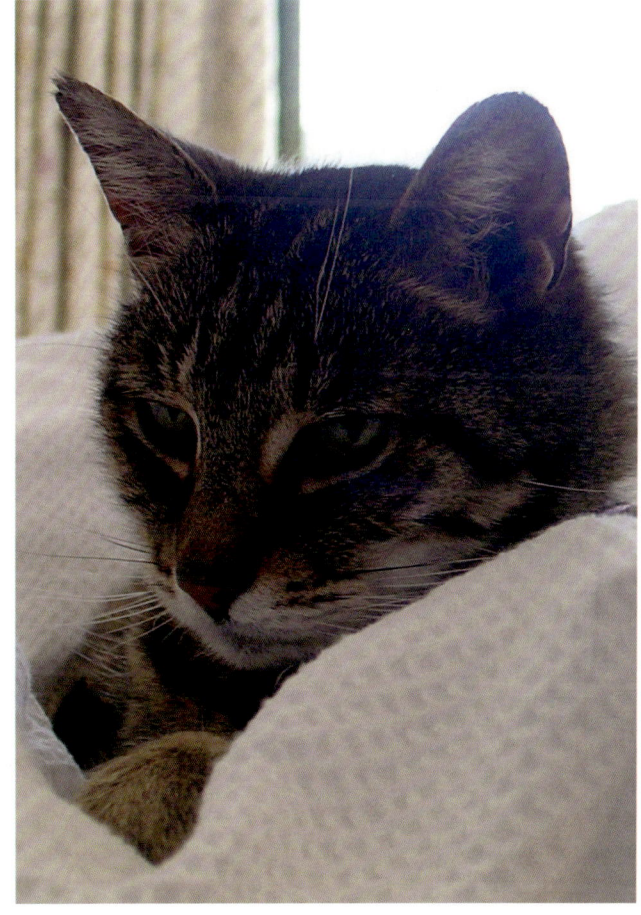

Important Legal Information:

Cat Professional has developed this book with reasonable skill and care to provide general information on feline health and care in relation to lower urinary tract disease. This book however does not, and cannot, provide advice on any individual situation. It is not a substitute for advice from a veterinary surgeon on each individual situation.

Cat Professional therefore strongly recommends that users seek, and follow, advice from their veterinary surgeon on any health or other care concerns that they may have concerning their cats. Users should not take, or omit to take, action concerning the health or care of their cats in reliance on the information contained in this book and so far as permissible by law, Cat Professional excludes all liability and responsibility for the consequences of any such action or omission in reliance on that information. While this book does not provide advice on, or recommend treatments or medications for, individual situations, users attention is brought to the fact that some of the medications referred to in this book may not be licensed (veterinary approved) in all countries and therefore may not be available in all countries.

SECTION 1 | the emotional side of things

Receiving bad news: coping with the emotional side of receiving a diagnosis of lower urinary tract disease in your cat

Being told that your cat has feline lower urinary tract disease (FLUTD) may have caused you some anxiety. FLUTD is a complex condition to understand and some cats with this condition need treatment for the rest of their life. This section will aim to reassure you as well as prepare you for what is to come.

By the time that a diagnosis of FLUTD has been made, many cats will have been suffering from constant or intermittent signs of their illness for some time. FLUTD is not only distressing for cats but also is one of the most stressful and worrying conditions for an owner to cope with.

What is wrong with my cat?

FLUTD is the veterinary term used to describe a number of illnesses that can affect the bladder and/or urethra of cats. Affected cats most commonly show signs including frequent urination (pollakiuria), passing bloody urine (haematuria), agitation or meowing when urinating, passing urine in inappropriate locations (e.g. outside the litter tray, referred to as periuria) and showing pain and/or difficulty passing urine (dysuria). Some cats with FLUTD will be presented to their vets because of behavioural changes such as apparent loss of house training, aggression and over-grooming of the belly. All of these are potential signs of FLUTD in your cat. Section 2 covers the scientific aspects of this condition in much greater detail – you can read about the causes of FLUTD, how vets diagnose the condition and how it can best be treated.

> **The overwhelming majority of cases of FLUTD are caused by medical conditions which are completely out of an owner's control i.e. your cat is not ill because of something you have done!**

Could I have prevented this from happening – was it my fault?

Many owners will immediately panic that they could have done more to prevent an illness from developing or that, if only they had taken their cat to the vet sooner, things might be different. Although it is impossible to generalise or comment specifically on an individual cat's circumstances, the following statements are usually true:

- The overwhelming majority of cases of FLUTD are caused by medical conditions which are completely out of an owner's control i.e. your cat is not ill because of something you have done!

- Although it is always advisable to take your cat to the vet as soon as you realise it is ill, in most situations a short delay is unlikely to have changed their chances of recovery. One important exception to this would be urethral obstruction (also referred to as a 'blocked' cat). This situation is always an emergency and treatment should be given as soon as it is suspected. Section 2 discusses this condition in more detail

SECTION 1 | the emotional side of things

What is the treatment for this disease?
Where possible, the cause of the FLUTD should be identified so that specific treatment can be given. For example, infections of the urine can be treated with a course of antibiotics and some bladder stones can be 'dissolved' by feeding a special prescription diet.

A range of additional treatments can help cats with idiopathic FLUTD – the most common type of FLUTD diagnosed in cats. This is discussed in more detail in Section 2.

If this is the first time that your cat has suffered from FLUTD then your vet may suggest that supportive or symptomatic treatments are used in the first instance. For example, a painkiller injection may be given to help your cat feel more comfortable. If the illness persists or worsens or if it recurs then further investigations are indicated to diagnose the cause of the FLUTD. This is discussed in more detail in Section 2.

Is my cat in pain?
FLUTD can be a very painful condition and this makes it distressing for both cat and owner. In cats with bladder stones, and other persistent problems, the discomfort associated with these continues until the stones have been treated. In cats with idiopathic FLUTD, the most common type of FLUTD, the affected cat typically suffers from 'episodes' of FLUTD. Each episode typically lasts for a few days. In between these episodes, the cat is apparently not in discomfort.

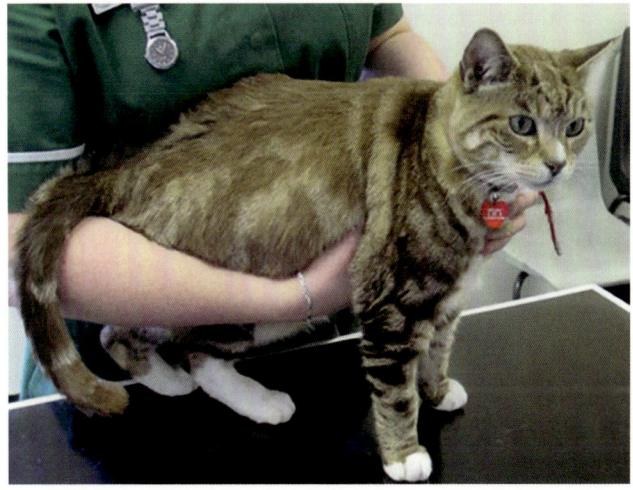

Is it fair to put my cat on lots of different medications – am I being cruel to treat it?
Not all cats with FLUTD need medication. For example, feeding a moist diet and encouraging your cat to drink more may be sufficient to manage this condition. If your cat has been prescribed medication and you are concerned about how you may be able to give this to your cat, then it may be helpful to hear that:

- Some cats are surprisingly easy to medicate
- Some cats will reliably eat treatments in their food

SECTION 1 | the emotional side of things

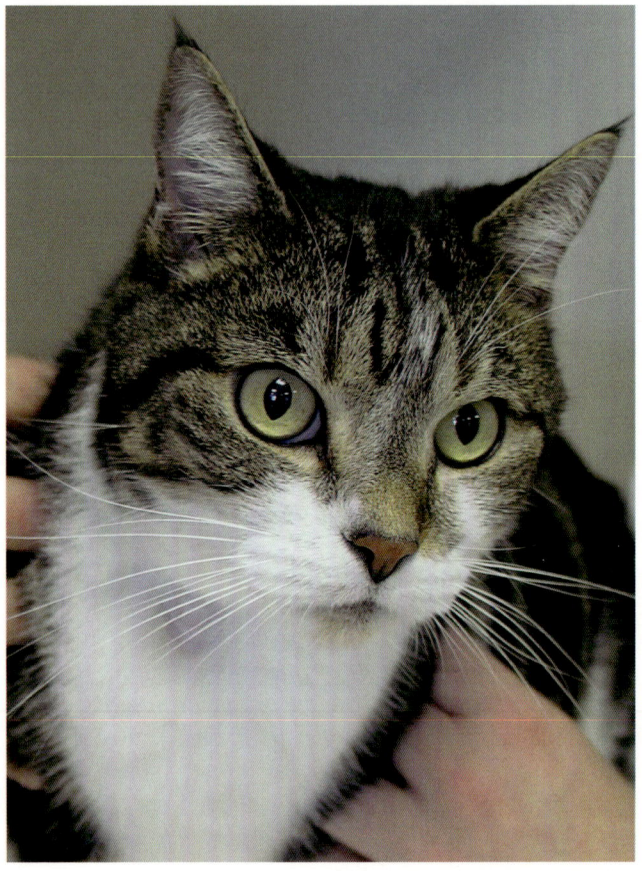

- For those cats on multiple medications empty gelatine capsules obtained from a vet or pharmacist can be very helpful. Several medicines can be put into one empty gelatine capsule reducing medication into one easy dosage

It may take some time for you, and your cat, to get used to all of the treatments your vet has suggested but as long as your cat is happy and coping, it is worthwhile persevering. Don't forget to discuss how treatment is going with your vet – if you are having problems, they may well have solutions or suggestions for you.

Also, remember that we are talking about your cat – no one knows your cat better than you and if you feel that the treatment suggested is not right, for whatever reason, then your vet should respect this.

I'm not sure I can cope with treating my cat – help!
Learning of a diagnosis of FLUTD may have come as a shock and will take some time to get used to. Once you have had a chance to think things through, chat with friends/family and your vet, hopefully everything will seem clearer and less daunting.

You can only do your best when it comes to caring for your cat and it is not always possible to do everything you want. For example if you have severe arthritis and are unable to give your cat a pill this may affect the level of treatment you can provide. Likewise, if your cat is completely intolerant to the thought of being medicated, this may prevent you from giving some treatments

SECTION 1 | the emotional side of things

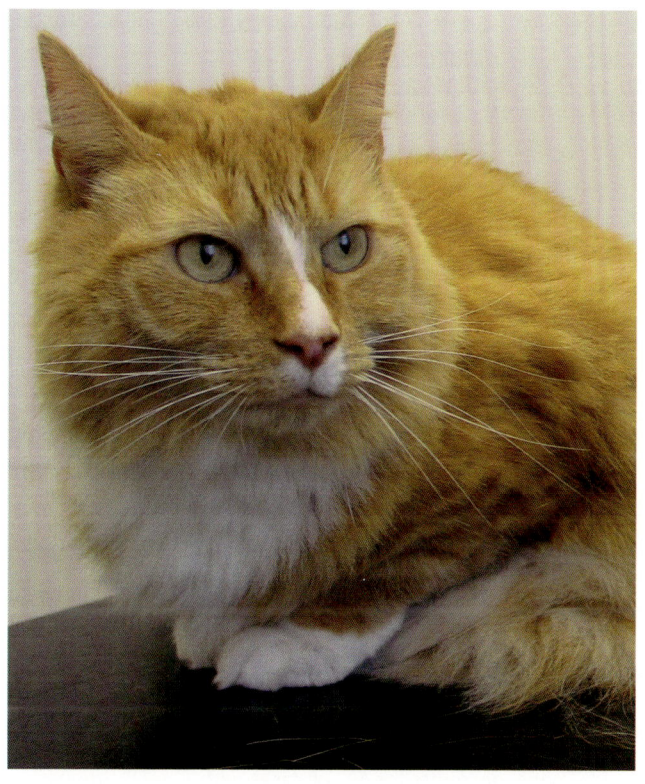

to it. In many situations, there are other options available – for example trying to hide medications in food or asking your vet to give an injection of the drug. Please note injections are not available for every type of medicine. In any case, your vet should be able to talk you through the options and, together, you should be able to make a plan that you both feel comfortable with.

Is FLUTD life-threatening?

This very much depends on the cause of the problem – for example a cat with urethral obstruction is in danger of dying within a matter of hours if left untreated, but many cats with idiopathic FLUTD can live a normal lifespan with this condition. If urethral obstruction is suspected – for example if your cat is straining and not passing any urine, or is known to have not urinated for more than 12 hours – then it is essential to take them to the vet as a matter of urgency. This is discussed in more detail in Section 2.

SECTION 2 | explaining the science of lower urinary tract disease

What is feline lower urinary tract disease (FLUTD)?

Feline lower urinary tract disease (FLUTD) is a term used to encompass a number of conditions which affect the bladder and urethra. Your vet may also refer to this condition as cystitis. The definition of cystitis is inflammation of the urinary bladder. The symptoms of FLUTD are very similar regardless of the cause. This is a condition which is most common in young and middle aged cats.

FLUTD is sub-divided into obstructive and non-obstructive. Obstructive is the term used to describe cats with urethral obstruction. Obstructed cats are unable to pass urine and are often presented to their vets because they have been repeatedly straining to urinate without success. A lay term for this is a 'blocked' cat.

Patients with non-obstructive disease remain able to pass urine. Typically, these cats will be straining to pass small quantities of urine on a frequent basis.

What is the urinary tract?

The urinary tract includes the organs involved in production of urine (the kidneys) and all of the structures involved in the transit of urine out of the body. This includes:

- The ureters: there are two of these – one for each of the kidneys. These tubes take urine from the kidneys to the bladder
- The bladder: this is where urine is stored prior to urination (micturition is the scientific name for urinating)
- The urethra: this is the tube which takes urine from the bladder to the outside

The term 'lower urinary tract' generally refers to the bladder and urethra. Thus lower urinary tract disease is illness affecting the bladder and urethra. Some other organs are closely involved with the lower urinary tract – in male cats this includes the prostate. In female cats, the urethra empties into the vagina.

What causes FLUTD?

There are several important causes of lower urinary tract disease in cats. The frequency of the different causes does vary according to the age group of the cats as will be discussed in each section below. The different causes of FLUTD can occur separately or in interacting combinations. For example, bacterial infections can occur in association with bladder stones.

1. Feline idiopathic cystitis (FIC) or idiopathic FLUTD (iFLUTD)
This is the most common cause of FLUTD in cats and is especially common in young and middle aged cats where it accounts for more than 50% of cases of FLUTD. In cats over 10 years of age, iFLUTD only accounts for 5% of cases with FLUTD. Idiopathic means 'cause unknown' so this category is one where all of the known causes of FLUTD have been ruled out. Affected cats often have several of the following factors in common:

- Overweight
- Lead a sedentary or very inactive lifestyle
- Indoor-only cats or have restricted access outdoors or dislike going outdoors

SECTION 2 | explaining the science of lower urinary tract disease

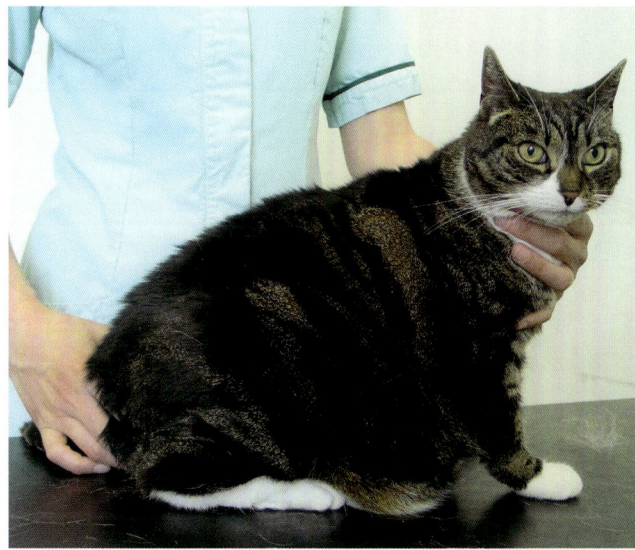

Cats that are overweight are more vulnerable to developing FLUTD.

- Use an indoor litter box

- Live in a multi-animal household. There is often tension between the FLUTD cat and other members of the household

- Neutered cats are more vulnerable than entire males (Toms) or entire females (Queens)

- Single cats living in indoor-only situations with little environmental enrichment are more vulnerable

- Cats that are very dependent on their owners and that suffer from separation anxiety are especially at risk of developing FLUTD

Persian and black and white domestic short haired cats may be over-represented with this condition and in countries with cold winters clinical signs may be seasonal being worse from Autumn to early Spring.

FIC can be obstructive or non-obstructive. Male cats are most vulnerable to obstructive disease and this needs emergency treatment.

Clinical signs with non-obstructive FIC are usually self-limiting – in other words, the cats get better on their own, usually within five to ten days. However, most affected cats suffer from repeated episodes of clinical signs which can be very distressing to both cat and owner. In general the frequency and severity of these episodes gradually decreases with time.

Unfortunately, in spite of more than 30 years of research, no one knows the precise cause of FIC. It has been suggested that this condition is similar to an illness called interstitial cystitis – an idiopathic bladder disease affecting people. A recent hypothesis suggested that FIC is a condition seen when 'a susceptible cat is placed in a provocative environment' and that disease results from changes in the cat's nervous and hormonal systems leading to an inability to cope with environmental stress. Affected cats are believed to suffer from defective information processing by their brain meaning that they are vulnerable to developing FIC when stressed. Genetic and/or developmental factors are thought to be very important in causing this problem. Genetic factors could account for the increased incidence of FIC in some families of cats. Stress in the peri-natal period (when the kitten is developing in the womb and during its first few weeks of life) is thought to cause abnormal development of the cat's stress

SECTION 2 | explaining the science of lower urinary tract disease

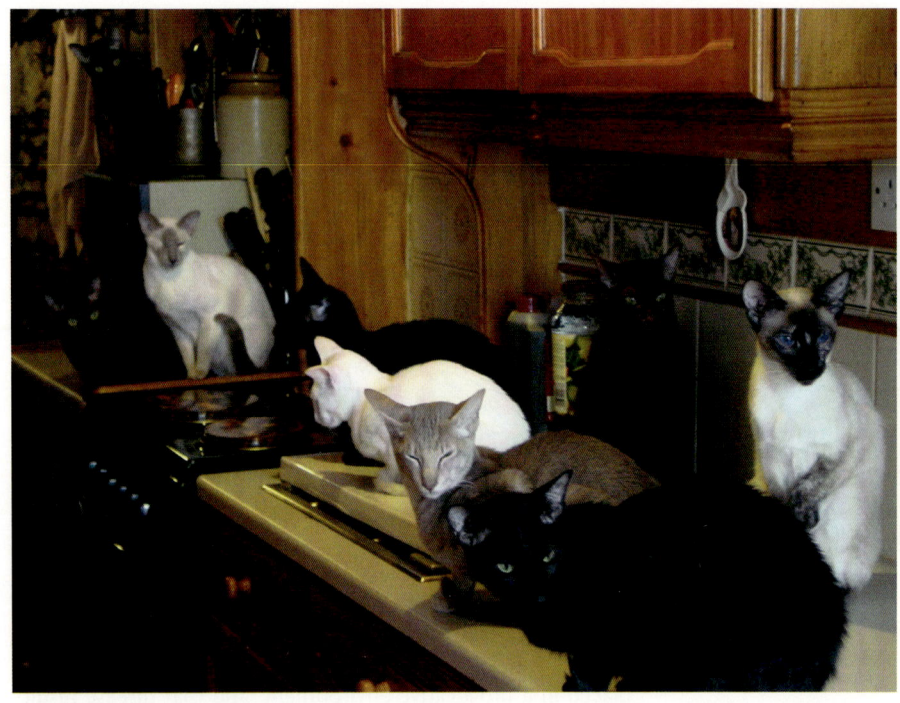

Cats living in multicat households are more likely to suffer from FLUTD – especially if there is tension between the cats.

management system. The end result is altered processing within the brain and nerve supply between this and the bladder. It is not clear whether these cats have an abnormal stress response system which predisposes them to negative effects of chronic stress (such as FIC) or whether being in a state of chronic stress leads to malfunctioning of the stress response system. This situation may be further worsened by changes to the protective glycosaminoglycan layer which lines the bladder. This lining protects the bladder cells from coming into contact with irritating substances which are normally present in the urine such as a salt called potassium.

Stress is believed to play a very important role in triggering and/or exacerbating FIC. Stress is defined as being 'acute' or 'chronic'. In medical terminology, acute means sudden (occurring over a period of up to a few days) whereas chronic conditions have been present for at least a couple of weeks. Causes of chronic stress and especially those which the cat has little or no control

SECTION 2 | explaining the science of lower urinary tract disease

over, are suggested to be the most damaging. Acute stress can also trigger FIC and this can include causes of stress which the cat is able to manage or evade through using normal coping strategies such as hiding.

Suggested stressors (causes of stress) include:

- Living in a multiple animal household, especially when there is conflict or tension between cats
- Moving house
- New additions to the house e.g. new cats, new babies
- Stress associated with urination – for example:
  – Competition for using a litter box affecting a cat's ability to access the litter box
  – Using a cat litter which the cat doesn't like. For example changing the cat litter from something which the cat has used for years
  – Placing the litter box in an unsuitable location. For example a litter box overlooked by cats outside the house or in a very busy part of the home
  – Providing a dirty litter box
  – Providing a litter box which is difficult for the cat to access. For example an arthritic cat may have difficulty getting into a high-sided box
- Sudden changes to the cat's diet
- Bad weather deterring a cat from going outside when it normally uses the outdoors to urinate

Owner stress can be transmitted to the cat and if the owner/cat bond is very close this can be very stressful for the cat.

- Other cats in the neighbourhood preventing a cat from going outdoors (or making life outdoors very stressful and unappealing)
- Building work in the house – especially if this affects core areas of the house such as the kitchen and areas where the cat spends a lot of its time
- Changes to the owner's schedule – for example working away from the home for longer periods, shift-working etc. Cats that are very 'needy' and dependent on their owners are especially vulnerable to stress associated with these changes
- Owner stress can also be transmitted to the cat and if the owner/cat bond is very close this can be very stressful for the cat. Often the combination of cat and owner stress exacerbates each other and worsens the situation

Reducing stress – especially causes of chronic stress – is therefore likely to be of great benefit to a cat suffering from FIC. Reducing stress should help to reduce the frequency and severity of bouts of FIC. Strategies for reducing stress in the home are discussed on pages 39-44.

Stress is thought to affect FIC cats in a different way to normal cats. Because of the changes in their nervous system and processing of information, they respond to stress by showing

SECTION 2 | explaining the science of lower urinary tract disease

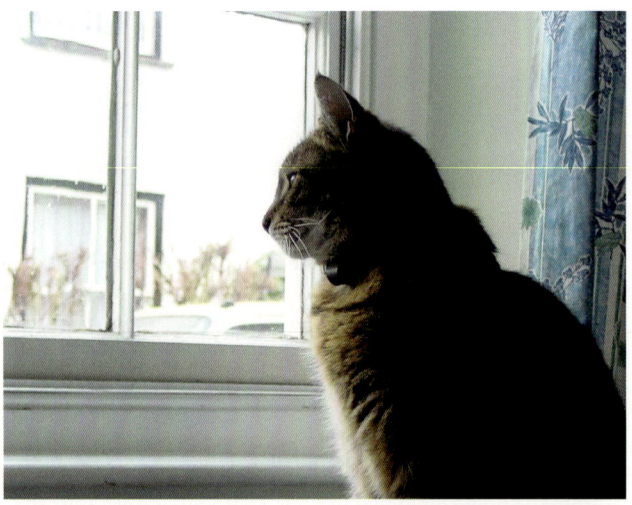

Indoor-only cats and cats with limited access outdoors are more likely to suffer from FLUTD.

more displacement activity. Displacement activity is defined as a behaviour performed out of its usual context and which is apparently irrelevant to the current situation – often occurring when in situations of stress or conflict. For FIC cats, the displacement activity might include eating and drinking more (so cats can be stress-eaters like some humans), over-grooming and urinating.

The compromised 'stress management' that FIC sufferers have means that it is vital to try and reduce causes of stress in the home. The home should be managed so that stress is at a minimum and the cat is free to express all of the normal feline behaviours that it wishes to. This will be discussed in more detail in the treatment section (especially pages 39-44).

So far, research has not shown that any bacterial, fungal or viral infection is consistently associated with FIC. However this is still an area of research since some infections are very difficult to diagnose.

Another area of research has been into the role that glycosaminoglycans have in cats with FIC. In all cats, a thin layer of glycosaminoglycans (GAGs) lines the internal surface of the bladder and is thought to help protect the bladder cells from noxious/irritating substances in the urine (such as acid, potassium, magnesium and calcium). The GAG layer also helps to stop bacteria and crystals in the urine from sticking to the bladder lining and causing problems. If the GAG lining is damaged or lost then this can allow these noxious substances to enter the bladder lining causing inflammation and stimulating the nerve supply to the bladder, resulting in sensation of pain.

Therefore, nerves within the bladder can be stimulated either by the brain (for example, in response to stress) or by 'local' triggers in the bladder (for example inflammation). When inflammation is triggered by the brain and nervous system, it is called 'neurogenic' inflammation.

2. Urolithiasis

Urolithiasis is the second possible cause of FLUTD to be discussed. Urolithiasis is the medical term for stones which are most commonly located in the bladder (cystic uroliths). Calculi is another word for uroliths which you may hear used. Stones can leave the bladder via the urethra. Small stones can be passed in the urine but larger stones can block the urethra causing urethral obstruction. Urethral obstruction is a life-threatening condition that needs urgent treatment.

SECTION 2 | explaining the science of lower urinary tract disease

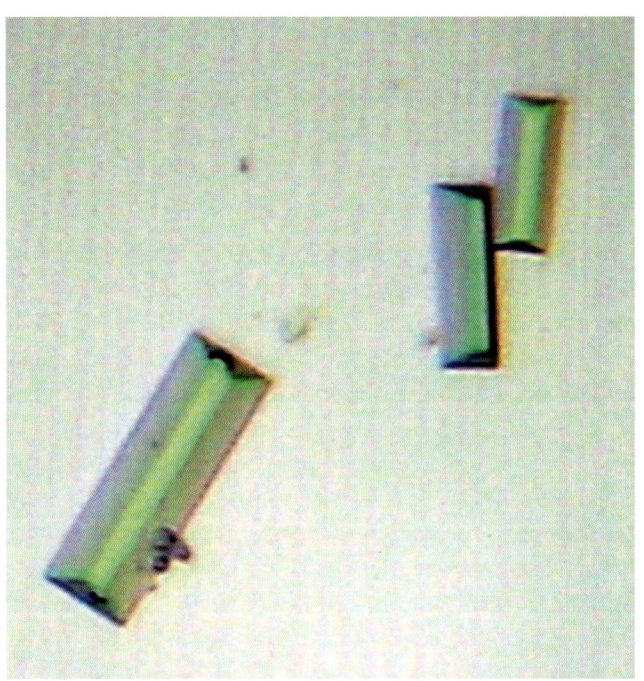

Crystals are only visible under the microscope and most healthy cats eating standard dry catfood will have crystals in their urine.

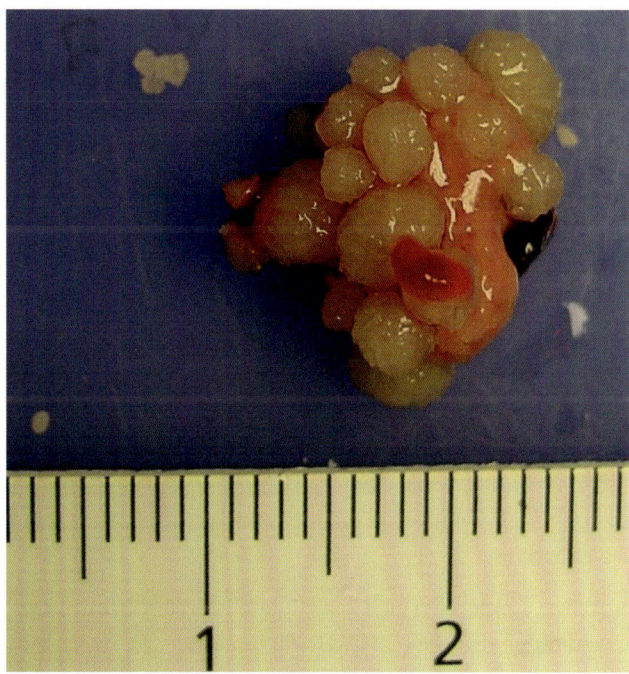

A cluster of stones removed surgically from a cat's bladder.

Uroliths are the cause of FLUTD in around 20% of cats less than 10 years of age and around 10% of cats older than 10 years of age. Uroliths can cause inflammation through irritating the lining of the bladder. There are several different types of bladder stones from which cats can suffer – common examples are struvite (also known as magnesium ammonium phosphate) and oxalate. Struvite stones used to be the most common stones seen in cats. Unfortunately, since diets were changed to make struvite stones less likely, calcium oxalate stones started to become more common. Certain breeds of cat are more vulnerable to oxalate stones – namely Persian and Ragdoll cats. Oxalate stones are also more common in cats with a condition called idiopathic hypercalcaemia (when the blood calcium levels are too high) and in older cats (because these cats tend to have more acidic urine which makes formation of these stones more likely).

SECTION 2 | explaining the science of lower urinary tract disease

It is important to know that stones are not the same as crystals.

Stones are visible to the naked eye and vary in appearance according to their make-up. Struvite stones tend to be very smooth and pebble-like in appearance. Oxalate stones are often very spiky and rough. It is not unusual to have a stone which has an outer structure of one type (e.g. oxalate) with a different internal structure (e.g. struvite).

Crystals are not visible to the naked eye and are only visible by looking down a microscope unless there are large numbers of crystals in which case a sandy or gritty appearance might be seen in a urine sample. Crystalluria, presence of crystals in the urine, is not damaging to the health and does not cause FLUTD. Most cats eating a standard dry diet will have crystals in their urine and this is normal. Crystals can be a cause of concern in a few situations:

- When a type of crystal called urate is seen this can be an indication that the cat has a liver problem
- When large numbers of crystals are seen, especially in situations where they form a sandy deposit visible to the naked eye, then this can increase the risk of obstruction
- In a cat with urolithiasis the type of crystal present may indicate the type of stone present. In other words, if crystals are found in the urine of a cat with a bladder stone then the crystal type is often the same as the stone type (for example struvite). However, this is not always true so cannot be relied upon

3. Urethral plugs

Urethral plugs are the third cause of FLUTD to be discussed. Urethral plugs account for about 20% of FLUTD cases in cats less than 10 years of age. Plugs are less common in older cats, accounting for around 6% of FLUTD cases in cats over the age of 10.

Urethral plugs are a potential cause of urethral obstruction which is a life-threatening condition. The plugs are made up of a protein matrix (a mixture of inflammatory proteins and mucus with cells and blood clots mixed in) with some crystals (usually struvite). The matrix is formed from protein which has leaked through the bladder wall as a result of inflammation of the bladder lining. Urethral plugs are often associated with FIC and most clinicians believe that this is a subset of FIC making FIC responsible for around 75% of cases of FLUTD in cats under the age of 10 years. Rarely urethral plugs can occur as a result of bladder stones, tumours or infections. The protein matrix can also cause a urethral obstruction even when no crystals are present. However, when crystals are present, these can become trapped in the matrix and make it more likely to cause an obstruction. Urethral obstruction can be caused by the plug itself but also can be caused by urethral spasm (tightening of the muscles around the urethra) associated with the pain caused by the presence of FIC and/or a plug.

4. Infections

Bacterial infection is a rare cause of FLUTD accounting for less than 2% of cases in cats less than 10 years of age. However, in older cats, bacterial infections are much more common,

SECTION 2 | explaining the science of lower urinary tract disease

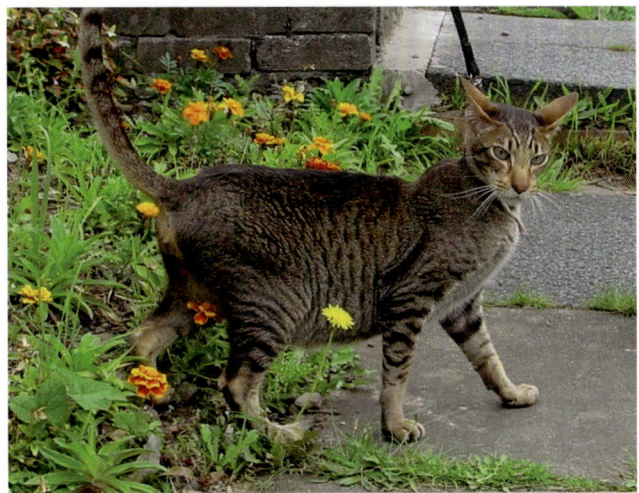

Some indoor cats appreciate access outdoors on a lead and may prefer to urinate and defecate outside if this is allowed.

accounting for around 45% of cases. This is thought to be the case since:

- Older cats often have more dilute urine which is easier for bacteria to grow in

- Older cats often have other illnesses which predispose them to infections for a variety of reasons. Common illnesses include diabetes mellitus ('sugar diabetes'), hyperthyroidism (an overactive thyroid gland) and kidney disease

Bacterial infections can be caused by passing a urinary catheter into the bladder, and cats with other bladder conditions (such as stones and tumours) are more vulnerable to becoming infected. The most common bacterial infections are *Escherichia coli* (*E.coli* – responsible for 40-70% of cases), *Enterococcus* species (responsible for 25-30% of cases) and *Staphylococcus* species (responsible for up to 20% of cases). Cats suffering from bacterial urinary tract infections (UTIs) are vulnerable to having repeated infections and for the infection to travel from the bladder to the kidneys – known as an 'ascending infection'. A bacterial infection of the kidneys is known as pyelonephritis and this can cause or worsen kidney disease.

Very rarely, fungal urinary tract infections can occur. These are usually seen in cats with severely impaired immune function – for example in a cat infected with feline immunodeficiency virus (FIV) or on anti-cancer treatment.

5. Other causes of FLUTD

Other less common causes of FLUTD include:

- Tumours – for example transitional cell carcinoma of the bladder. This is a rare, malignant tumour of the bladder that can affect older cats in particular

- Traumatic damage – for example as a consequence of a road traffic accident there may be bleeding into the urine

- Incontinence – this is rare in cats and can occur for a variety of reasons including:

    – Congenital anatomical abnormalities such as ectopic ureters (ureters which bypass the bladder to exit in the urethra for example). Congenital means present from birth

    – Disease or damage to the nerve supply to the bladder – for example following a road traffic accident or cancer which damages the spine

    – Following surgery to the urinary tract

SECTION 2 | explaining the science of lower urinary tract disease

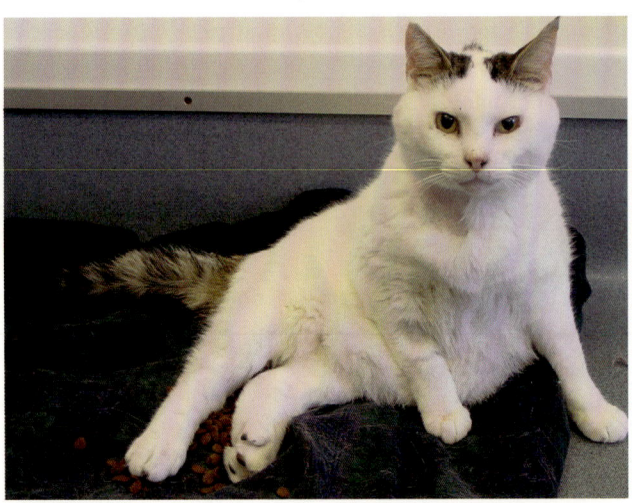

This cat has suffered from spinal trauma as a result of a car accident and is suffering from incontinence due to a damaged nerve supply to the bladder.

- As part of a dysautonomia (a condition which used to be referred to as Key-Gaskell Syndrome). This condition often also affects other organs so clinical signs might include mydriasis (dilation of the pupils), reduced tear production, dry mouth, slow heart rate and regurgitation of food

- Rarely, urinary tract infections can cause incontinence

6. Behavioural causes of FLUTD
In some cases, the cause of the FLUTD signs is the result of a purely behavioural problem. In some of these cats, a physical disease was present in the past and this probably contributed to the recurrence of signs. Stress management (see pages 39-44) is of particular importance in the treatment of these cats.

What is periuria?

Periuria is the medical term for urinating in inappropriate places rather than the litter box or garden. Common locations for periuria include carpet, duvets, sofas, baths, sinks and plastic bags. Causes of periuria include:

- FLUTD

- Behavioural problems – for example an unwillingness to use a litter tray due to conflict with another cat or fear of the litter tray

- A reluctance to use the litter tray due to a dislike of the litter used (some cats will perch on the sides of the tray!)

- Disruption to the normal places where the cat urinates – for example moving the litter tray to another location or building an extension over your cat's favourite flower bed

- Cats suffering from an excessive thirst (polydipsia) – for example due to kidney disease – which means that they have an increased need to pass urine (polyuria). If they cannot get to an appropriate place in time, affected cats may choose an inappropriate location

- Cats suffering from arthritis or other problems affecting their mobility and hence their ability to climb into an appropriate place or use a cat-flap to get outside for example

- Cats trapped in a room and unable to get to their litter tray or cat-flap

'Spraying' – depositing urine as a scent signal – should be distinguished from periuria. To spray urine, the cat stands up, spraying a small amount of urine onto the vertical surface

SECTION 2 | explaining the science of lower urinary tract disease

behind it. This differs from urination where the cat squats to pass urine onto a horizontal surface. Common locations for spraying include doors, windows, the area by the cat-flap and electrical equipment. It is worth noting that some male cats suffering from urethral pain associated with their FLUTD may choose to urinate in a standing position. They will usually pass more urine than occurs with spraying.

If your cat urinates in an inappropriate location, it is essential that the affected area is cleaned properly. If this is not done, the smell of the urine may encourage your cat to think that the area used is an appropriate place to use again. To clean the affected area:

- Wash with a biological or enzymatic washing powder that will break down the scent-marking chemicals in the urine

- Rinse with cold water and allow to dry

- Spray the area with surgical spirit (surgical alcohol) – for example, using a plant mister – then scrub and leave to dry. The alcohol helps to destroy the scent-marking chemicals present in the urine

Consider using specifically designed pet urine odour removal products (often available from veterinary clinics or large pet stores) to remove any residual smells.

If your cat has urinated on delicate fabrics then you may wish to test a small area first or initially use a less aggressive cleaning protocol. In addition to cleaning the affected area, where possible, prevent your cat from access to this area – for example by moving furniture or stopping the cat from going into the room concerned.

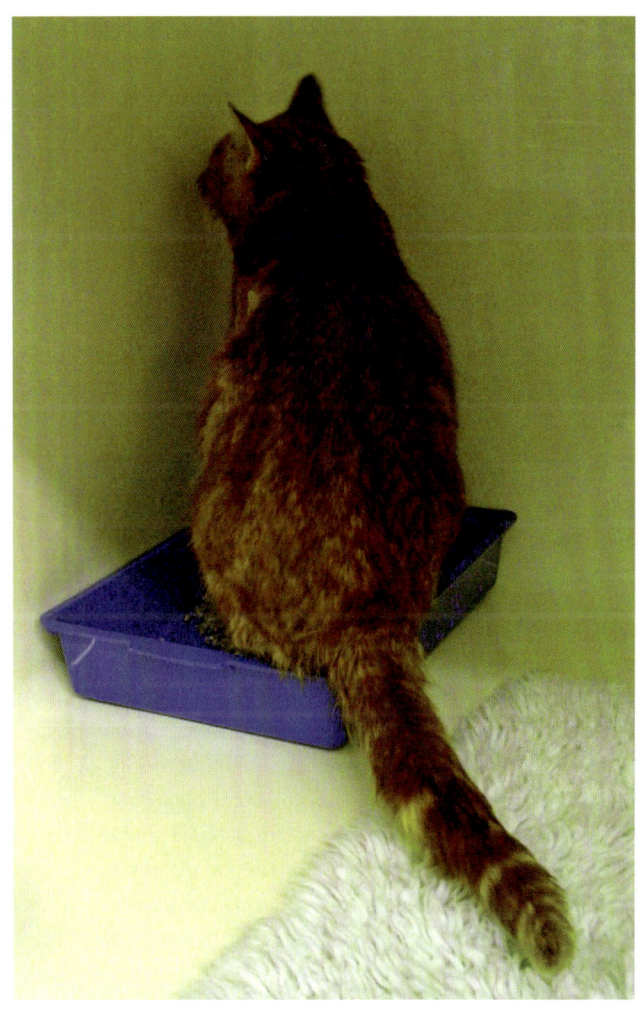

Unproductive straining to pass urine is a cause for immediate concern. Urethral obstruction can be rapidly fatal if left untreated.

SECTION 2 | explaining the science of lower urinary tract disease

International Cat Care's leaflet on spraying and soiling indoors (http://www.icatcare.org/advice/problem-behaviour/urine-spraying-cats) contains a lot of information and guidance on treating periuria.

What causes urethral obstruction?

Urethral obstruction can be caused by many different problems including:

- Problems affecting the urethra – for example urethral spasm (especially in FIC cats), urethral plugs, urolithiasis (stones), cancer, strictures (narrowing of the urethra) and prostate problems (very rare in cats)

- Problems affecting the bladder – for example FIC, urolithiasis (stones) and cancer

Obstruction is a very serious, potentially life-threatening condition. Accumulation of urine in the bladder causes a build up of substances normally excreted from the body. Affected cats commonly attempt to pass urine frequently but are unable to pass any urine at all. This is in contrast to cats with non-obstructive FLUTD where, typically, small amounts of urine are passed frequently. If signs of urethral obstruction persist for more than a few hours, the cat can become very ill and die. Other signs that might indicate obstruction include listlessness and weakness, loss of appetite, vomiting, development of an enlarged, hard and painful bladder which you might notice when the cat is picked up for example.

If urinary tract obstruction is suspected, the cat should receive immediate treatment from a veterinary surgeon. Rupture of the urinary tract, for example as a result of a road traffic accident, can cause the same blood disturbances and is just as life-threatening as urethral obstruction.

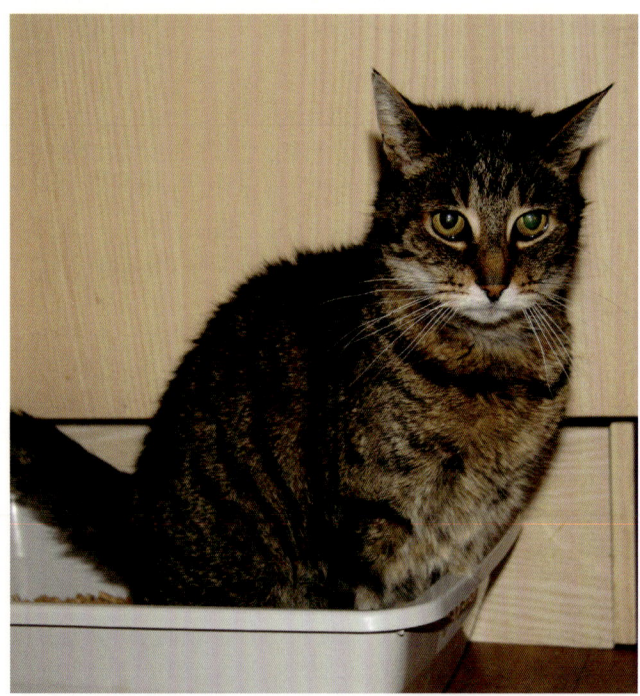

Straining to pass urine, frequent urination and showing signs of pain or discomfort are all signs of FLUTD.

SECTION 2 | explaining the science of lower urinary tract disease

Can FLUTD be prevented?

This is a difficult question to answer! Not all cats will be vulnerable to development of FLUTD but in those that are, the risk can be reduced by:

- Encouraging the cat to drink using tactics discussed later in this book
- Feeding a specifically designed diet rather than standard catfood
- Ensuring that the home is free from stress and that the cat is free to express their normal behaviour

All of these issues are discussed in more detail in the treatment section: How is FLUTD treated – especially in the section dealing with FIC (especially pages 38-47).

How can I tell if my cat is stressed?

It is not always easy to judge if your cat is stressed and different cats will respond to stress in different ways meaning that not all of the signs of stress will be seen in all individuals. Clues of stress include:

- Eating less, grooming less and becoming withdrawn. Please note that some cats – like some people – eat more when they are stressed!
- Not interacting with people and other pets – for example not wishing to play or go outside
- Showing signs of defensive aggression such as hissing at people or other pets in the home
- Urinating and defecating in inappropriate locations
- Over-grooming and self-mutilation can be seen in some cases

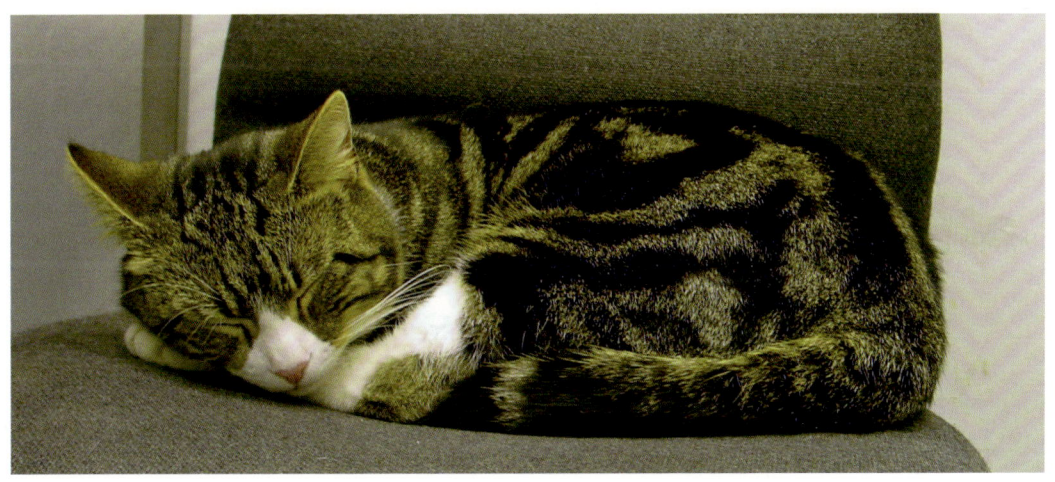

Feigning sleep (pretending to be asleep) can be a sign of stress, as in this patient at a veterinary clinic.

SECTION 2 | explaining the science of lower urinary tract disease

What are the signs of FLUTD?

The clinical signs of FLUTD commonly include:

- Difficult urination – for example straining to pass a very small amount of urine (dysuria)

- Increased frequency of urination – for example passing urine every few minutes (pollakiuria)

- Passing red urine which may contain blood clots (haematuria)

- Showing signs of pain – for example becoming agitated or restless, vocalising

- Knowingly passing urine in inappropriate places – for example on the kitchen floor or in the bath (periuria)

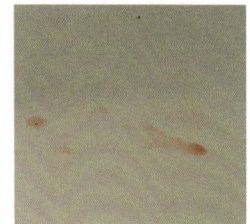

Passing small amounts of bloody urine is a common sign of FLUTD.

Other signs which can be seen include:

- Behavioural changes such as aggression and irritability with people and other animals

- Excessive grooming of the hair on the belly and perineum (area adjacent to the anus and where the urethra exits). This problem can also extend to include the skin on the inside of the back legs. Excessive grooming can cause hair-loss in these areas. The over-grooming is thought to be in response to pain in the bladder and/or urethra

- Evidence of urethral obstruction – a 'blocked' cat – for example straining and passing no urine. If this situation persists for more than a few hours, the cat can become very ill and die. Other signs that might indicate obstruction include listlessness and weakness, loss of appetite, vomiting, development of an enlarged, hard and painful bladder (which you might notice when the cat is picked up for example)

- Owners may see their cat straining and think that this is due to constipation rather than urinary problems

Unfortunately, these signs rarely indicate the precise cause of the FLUTD and, in fact, the most common cause of FLUTD is idiopathic disease. Idiopathic is the medical term for an illness where the cause is not known. To make a diagnosis of idiopathic FLUTD, all of the known causes of FLUTD need to be ruled out.

How is FLUTD diagnosed?

Lower urinary tract disease is often suspected on the basis of a history – for example when an owner reports that their cat is frequently squatting and straining to pass small amounts of bloody urine. If this is the first occasion on which your cat has had FLUTD then your vet may elect to treat it symptomatically without making a specific diagnosis. In other words, your vet may prescribe treatment which is likely to help the clinical signs such as a painkiller injection. If, however, your cat has had repeated bouts of FLUTD then it is likely that your vet will recommend that further tests are done to try and find the cause of the problem.

Investigations are therefore aimed at finding a specific diagnosis such as infections, tumours (cancers), bladder stones etc. In these cats, specific treatment of the problem identified will provide

SECTION 2 | explaining the science of lower urinary tract disease

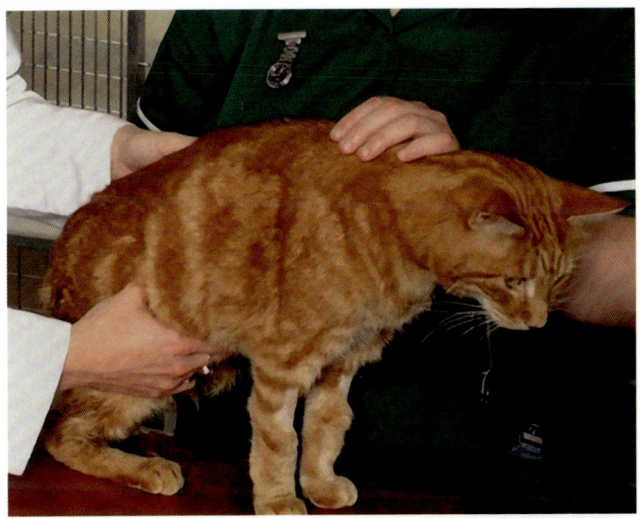

Assessing the size of the bladder is very important: a 'blocked' cat has a large bladder whereas other cats with FLUTD usually have a small, empty bladder.

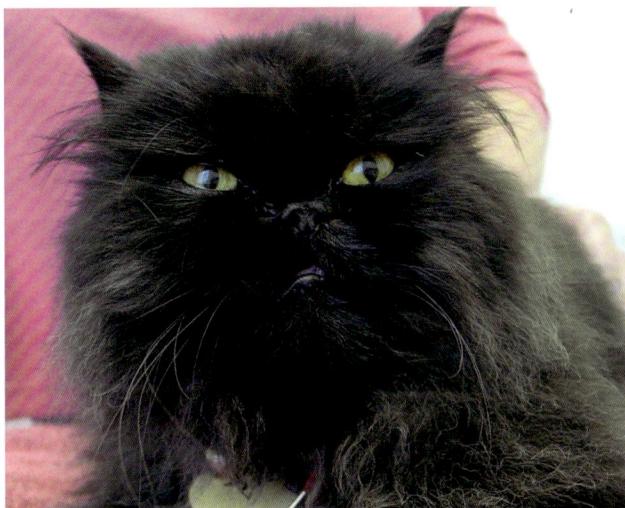

Persian cats are predisposed to FIC.

the best chance of a cure, or at least of long-term management. In those cats where the test results fail to find a specific cause, a diagnosis of FIC is made.

Appropriate diagnostic tests include:

- Taking a detailed patient history: this is important to gather as many clues as possible to the cause of the problem. For example, bladder cancer is most common in older cats and usually causes severe clinical signs. Cats with a painful urethra may be reported to be urinating in a different posture – they often pass small volumes of urine whilst standing more upright rather than squatting. Identifying chronic stress suffered by the cat is of particular importance in the diagnosis of FIC – for example history taking might reveal that the problem started or was exacerbated by the arrival of a new cat in the household or neighbourhood. As discussed later in the treatment of FIC section, it can be helpful to consult a veterinary behaviourist or other suitably qualified behavioural expert to discuss what stressors may be present in your household.

Certain conditions are more common in certain cats – for example FIC is most common in overweight, male neutered cats, often of a nervous disposition that are living in a multi-cat (or multi-animal) household. Persian cats are predisposed to both FIC and to oxalate urolithiasis.

- Physical examination: your vet will examine your cat to try and determine the cause of the FLUTD. Of major importance is identifying whether the bladder is small or large. A large,

SECTION 2 | explaining the science of lower urinary tract disease

hard, painful bladder is indicative of urethral obstruction (a 'blocked' cat).

A physical examination also helps to identify concurrent illnesses or other clues – for example a paralysed tail is present in some cases of spinal injury which might also be causing incontinence

- Blood tests: haematology and biochemistry tests are especially helpful in cats with urethral obstruction where life-threatening changes such as hyperkalaemia (high blood potassium levels) can be seen and need to be treated promptly. Blood tests are generally not helpful in diagnosing the cause of FLUTD in non-obstructive cases but may be recommended by your vet since they can give important clues such as hypercalcaemia (high blood calcium levels) in cats with oxalate bladder stones or anaemia (a shortage of red blood cells) due to chronic blood loss. Blood tests are also useful at identifying other indications of ill health such as dehydration or diabetes mellitus ('sugar diabetes').

Collection of blood samples should not be a stressful event for a cat. Blood is most easily collected from the jugular vein which is the largest vein and is located in the cat's neck. Alternatively blood can be collected from a cephalic vein which is a smaller vein, found on the front surface of the forelimbs.

Different laboratories have different reference ranges for blood test values and, different countries use different units which further confuses matters. The two types of unit measurements used are:

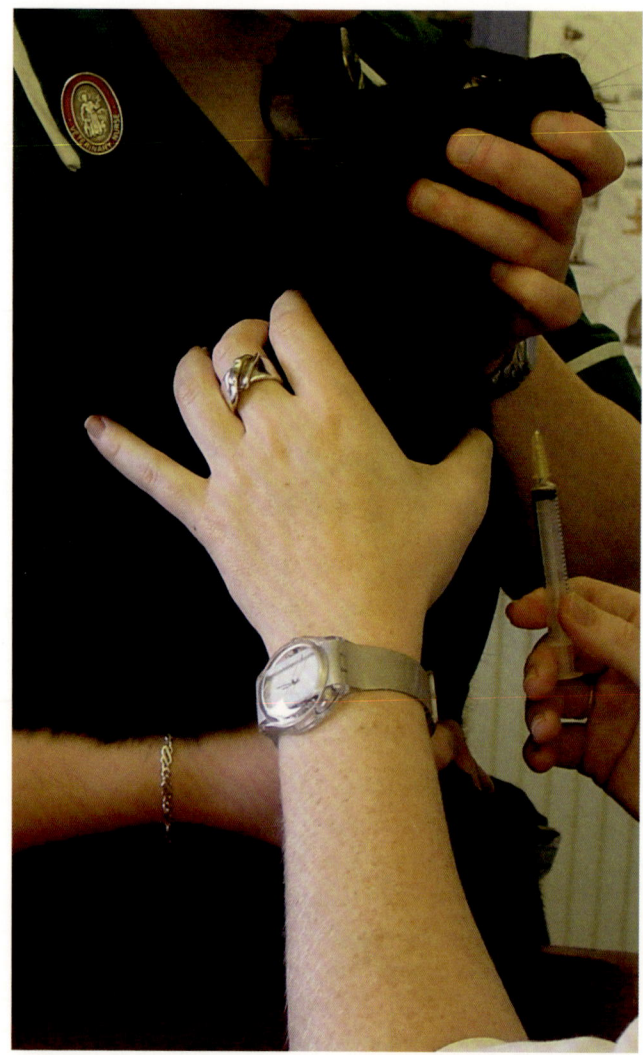

Collecting blood from the jugular vein should not be a stressful event for a cat

SECTION 2 | explaining the science of lower urinary tract disease

- Conventional units: mg/dl or mEq/l
- SI units: most widely used; mmol/l, g/l

The table below gives a guide to the reference range levels which are likely to be normal for where you live.

Parameter	'Typical reference range' – Conventional units	'Typical reference range' – SI units
Urea	17 – 29 mg/dl	6 – 10.5 mmol/l
Creatinine	< 2 mg/dl	< 175 µmol/l
Phosphate	2.9 – 6.0 mg/dl	0.95 – 1.95 mmol/l
Potassium	4.0 – 5.0 mEq/l	4.00 – 5.00 mmol/l
Sodium	145 – 157 mEq/l	145 – 157 mmol/l
Calcium	8 – 10 mg/dl	2.0 – 2.5 mmol/l
Albumin	2.4 – 3.9 mg/dl	24 – 39 g/l
Globulin	2.5 – 5.5 mg/dl	25 – 55 g/l
Total Protein	5.4 – 7.8 mg/dl	54 – 78 g/l
Bicarbonate	18 – 24 mEq/l	18 – 24 mmol/l
Packed cell volume (PCV) or haematocrit	28 – 45%	0.28 – 0.45
Haemoglobin	0.8 – 1.5 mg/dl	8 – 15 g/l

N.B. the reference range will vary slightly between laboratories so the following is just a rough guide:

mg/dl – milligrams per decilitre	µmol/l – micromoles per litre	g/dl – grams per decilitre
mmol/l – millimoles per litre	mEq/l – milliequivalents per litre	g/l – grams per litre.

A table with conversion factors for transforming SI units to Conventional units (and vice versa) is contained in the Reference section (Section 5).

SECTION 2 | explaining the science of lower urinary tract disease

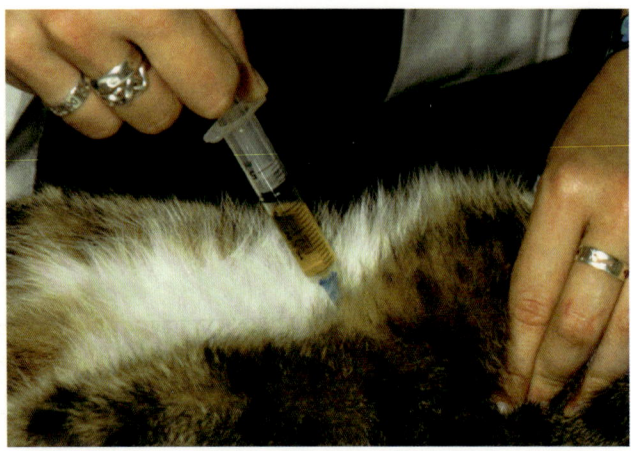

Collection of urine via a needle and syringe is the standard method for urine sample collection in cats. This cat is lying on his back (back legs on the left of the image) while the sample is collected.

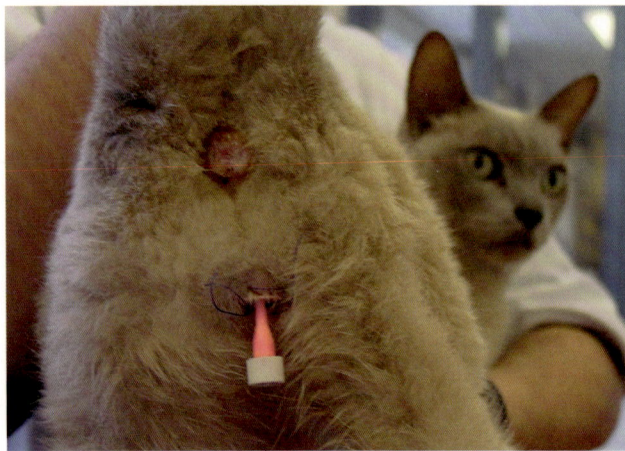

Urinary catheters can be used to collect urine samples from patients. This patient had a catheter placed to treat his urethral obstruction. The catheter is stitched to his skin and is plugged to stop urine dripping out.

4. Urinalysis: analysis of a urine sample is very helpful in cats with FLUTD.

Urine samples can be collected in a variety of ways:

- Cystocentesis: this is the procedure by which urine is collected using a needle and syringe. The cat is gently held and the needle is passed through the skin of the tummy into the bladder. This is not a painful procedure and allows collection of a sterile (free from bacterial contamination) sample which is ideal for the tests needed.

  In 'blocked' cats, cystocentesis is sometimes required to relieve the bladder distension. In these cats, cystocentesis can be uncomfortable since the bladder is so full. If the blockage is not relieved quickly, the bladder can also become very fragile and damaged because of being over-stretched. Cystocentesis in this situation carries a small risk of worsening this damage and potentially causing rupture (bursting) of the bladder.

- **Catheter samples**: urine can be collected using a catheter which is passed through the urethra (the tube from the outside of the cat to the bladder). Unfortunately this is not an appropriate technique for urine collection in most cats as it requires sedation (providing a state of calm and muscle relaxation using drugs) or anaesthesia (providing a state of unconsciousness, muscle relaxation and loss of pain sensation using certain drugs). In 'blocked' cats (cats with urethral obstruction) placing a catheter is often required as part of the treatment in which case this is an appropriate method for collecting a urine sample from the cat. Catheters are also often placed in cats having x-ray studies of their bladders and in this situation, this can be an appropriate method for collecting a urine sample

SECTION 2 | explaining the science of lower urinary tract disease

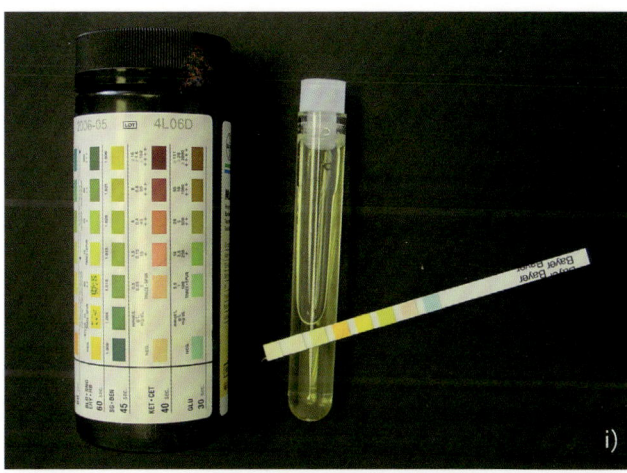

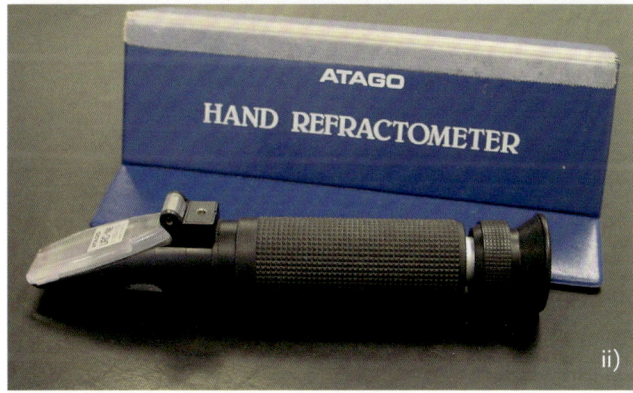

Urine is analysed in a number of ways including:

i) 'Dipstick' tests (as in people to detect sugar and protein in the urine).

ii) Urine concentration using a refractometer. Cats with FLUTD often have a specific gravity of greater than 1.045.

- **Free catch samples**: urine can be collected from an empty litter tray or one containing non-absorbent cat litter. Lots of different types of non-absorbant cat litter are available from your veterinarian or alternatives can be used (e.g. clean aquarium gravel, chopped up plastic bags). Once the cat has urinated, the urine can be collected using a syringe or pipette. It is important that the sample is collected as soon as possible after urination. Free catch samples are acceptable for initial assessment. For example the refractometer test which determines the concentration of the urine is not affected by the method of collection. Unfortunately, free catch samples are not ideal for bacterial culture or sediment examination as they will be contaminated by bacteria and debris in the litter tray and on the cat's paws. Where possible a cystocentesis sample is best for bacterial culture and sediment examination.

Urine should be analysed as quickly as possible. Important urine tests in a cat with FLUTD include:

– Assessment of the colour and cloudiness (turbidity): Normal urine is yellow and clear. Very concentrated urine can appear brown; presence of blood results in a pink to red discolouration (depending on the severity of the bleeding). If there are a lot of cells and protein (for example with inflammatory conditions), the urine can appear very cloudy

– Specific gravity measurement: A refractometer measures the urine specific gravity. Water has a specific gravity of 1.000. Normal cats usually produce urine with a specific gravity of at least 1.040. The lower the specific gravity, the more dilute the urine is. Cats with FLUTD often have very concentrated urine with a specific gravity of 1.045 or more. Most refractometers only measure to 1.050 so if the urine

SECTION 2 | explaining the science of lower urinary tract disease

is more concentrated than this, the result will be reported as 'greater than 1.050'

– Urine dipstick to check for sugar (glucose), assess the acidity of the urine (urine pH) and look for other abnormalities. Most cats with FLUTD will have acidic urine (pH less than 7) and since it is concentrated, the protein result on the dipstick may be increased (normally recorded as + or ++). Dipsticks have been designed for use with human urine so are not always as reliable when used with cat urine

– Sediment examination: This involves microscopic examination of a urine sample for red and white blood cells, bacteria, crystals or other material. For example this can help to diagnose a urinary tract infection. Crystals are a normal finding in cat urine, especially if the cat is fed a standard dry diet and also if the sample is not analysed immediately. As the temperature of urine cools (either at room temperature or in a refrigerator) crystals will form so their significance should not be over-estimated

– Bacterial culture to see whether there is any evidence of infection. Ideally this test should be performed on urine collected by cystocentesis. When a bacterial infection is diagnosed by the laboratory they will do a sensitivity test to identify which antibiotics are likely to be most effective in treating the infection. This is a test which takes a few days to perform

5. Diagnostic imaging

Diagnostic imaging is the term that refers to imaging techniques such as radiography (x-rays) and ultrasound. X-rays can be helpful in showing stones present in the kidneys, ureters,

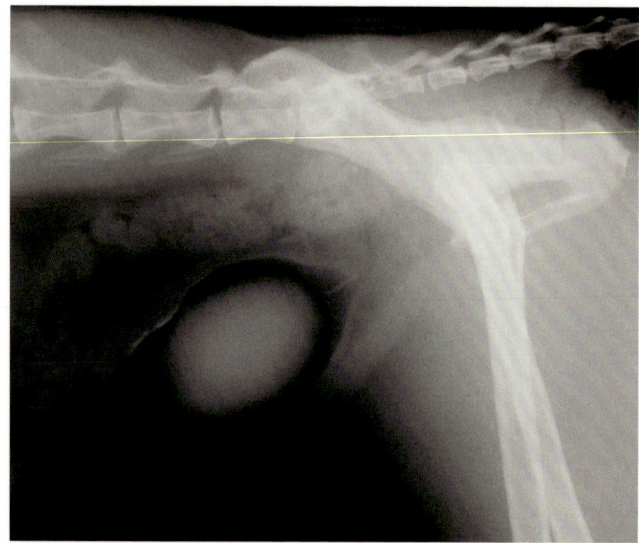

X-rays of the abdomen can be useful in finding thickened bladders. This image is from a cat with a bladder tumour. The bladder wall is thickened and very irregular. Contrast material has been injected into the bladder via a urethral catheter and shows as a white pool in the centre of the bladder. The bladder wall is thickened and very irregular especially from the 9 o'clock to 12 o'clock positions.

bladder and urethra. Not all stones will be visible on a standard 'plain' radiograph and this is one of the reasons for performing a contrast radiography study. Contrast radiographic studies necessitate anaesthesia. A retrograde contrast bladder study is most commonly performed and this involves draining the bladder of urine via a catheter placed in the urethra. Contrast material is then injected into the bladder using the catheter. The contrast material is a liquid which shows bright white on an x-ray. When the bladder is full of contrast material a radiograph is taken – this is called a positive contrast radiograph. After this

SECTION 2 | explaining the science of lower urinary tract disease

image has been taken, the contrast material is removed and air or carbon dioxide injected in its place. A further radiograph is taken – this is called a double contrast radiograph. Contrast radiographs are very good at showing uroliths, bladder thickening (common in FIC cases), bladder polyps and tumours. Positive contrast images of the urethra may be done (called a retrograde urethrogram) and are a good way of showing uroliths and strictures (narrowing of the urethra).

Ultrasound of the bladder can be helpful in finding stones, blood clots, thickening of the bladder wall, tumours and polyps. Ultrasound does not require sedation or anaesthesia and therefore is classed as a 'non-invasive' test. Unfortunately ultrasound is not able to visualise the full length of the urethra which is important in cats with FLUTD.

What other tests are helpful in cats with FLUTD?

Cystoscopy: This technique, available in some veterinary hospitals, involves passing a small endoscope (camera) through the urethra and into the bladder. This technique is helpful in examining the lining of the bladder for masses (e.g. tumours, polyps), areas of ulceration and areas of bleeding (often referred to as 'glomerulations', common in FIC cases).

Biopsy and cytology: in some cases, such as bladder tumours, collection of a sample of cells (cytology) or tissue (biopsy) is required to confirm the diagnosis. Both of these procedures require anaesthesia to perform. Cytology samples can be collected using a urinary catheter to suck a sample of cells out (a so-called suction biopsy or suction aspirate). A full thickness biopsy of the bladder requires abdominal surgery.

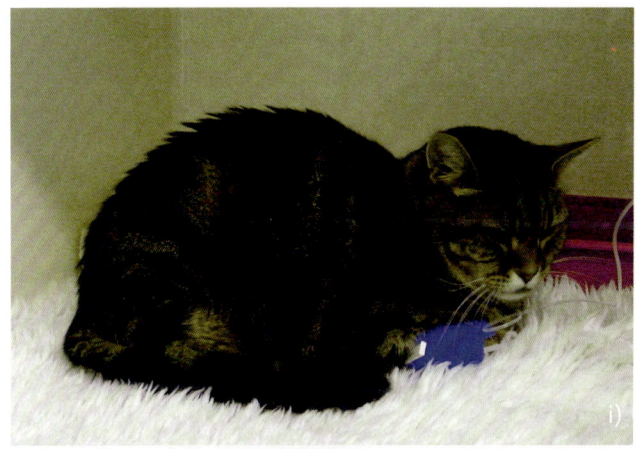

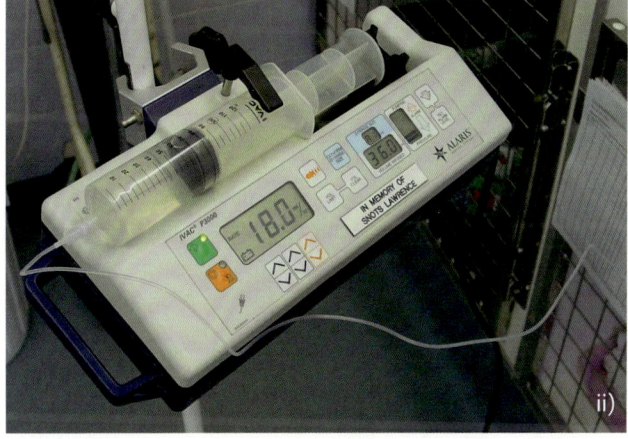

'Blocked' cats are usually dehydrated and need treatment with intravenous fluids (fluid given by a drip into a vein).

i. This involves placing a catheter (a tube) into the vein in the front leg. Drip tubing is attached to this.

ii. The fluid can be pumped into the cat using special pumps (such as the syringe pump shown in this picture) or with the aid of gravity.

SECTION 2 | explaining the science of lower urinary tract disease

Rectal examination: this can be especially helpful in cats with urethral obstruction where an enlarged prostate, stones, swelling and tumours may be detected.

In some cats, all of the results of diagnostic tests are normal. In these patients, it is possible that a purely behavioural problem exists. Another possibility is that the tests have been done when the cat is well. If this is the case then it might be helpful to repeat the tests at a time when signs of FLUTD are present.

How is FLUTD treated?

Successful treatment depends on having an accurate diagnosis. Therefore if signs of FLUTD are persistent or recur in spite of treatment, further investigations (as outlined above) are indicated. Where no underlying cause can be identified, a diagnosis of FIC is made.

1. **Treatment of cats with** urethral obstruction **– 'blocked' cats**

Urethral obstruction is a very serious condition which can result in the death of a cat within hours. Accumulation of urine in the bladder causes a build up of substances normally excreted from the body. This includes the protein breakdown products urea and creatinine, potassium and phosphate. A build up of urea and creatinine in the blood is referred to as 'azotaemia'. Affected cats are vulnerable to developing acidosis where the blood is more acidic than it should be. All of these consequences are very serious and can kill within hours. Rupture of the urinary tract, for example as a result of a road traffic accident, can cause the same blood disturbances and is just as life-threatening as urethral obstruction.

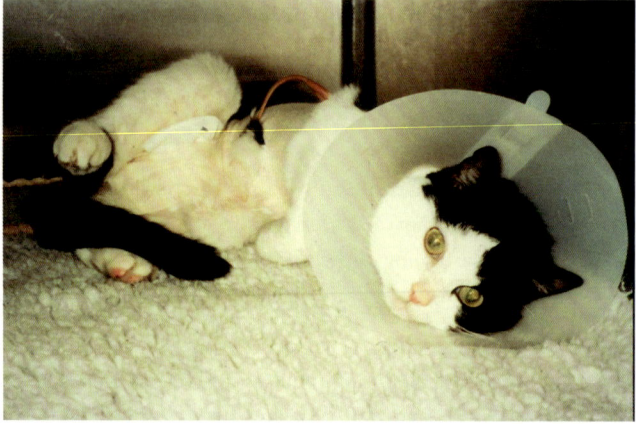

Jack, a cat who has had a tube cystotomy performed as part of his treatment for urethral obstruction. A tube emptying urine from his bladder passes through the skin of his tummy to the outside.

Before doing anything else, it is important to stabilise the cat so that they can safely undergo sedation or anaesthesia to treat their obstruction or rupture. The most common and serious complications are:

- Hyperkalaemia: This is the medical term for high blood potassium levels. Dangerously high blood levels of potassium can develop as a consequence of the obstruction. If untreated, this slows the heart eventually causing death. Hyperkalaemia is diagnosed by measuring blood potassium levels. If suitable facilities are not available to do this then other tests which can help include measuring the heart rate and performing an electrocardiogram (an ECG) which often shows clues of hyperkalaemia such as a slow heart rate, wide QRS complexes and tall T waves.

SECTION 2 | explaining the science of lower urinary tract disease

Treatment varies according to the severity of the hyperkalaemia. In mild cases, intravenous fluids (placing your cat on a drip) is very effective in lowering potassium levels as long as the urethral obstruction can be relieved. In severe cases, treatment required can include glucose and insulin. These treatments help to reduce the blood potassium levels by encouraging potassium to move out of the bloodstream and into cells. Calcium gluconate may be given to protect the heart from the life-threatening consequences of hyperkalaemia

- Acidosis: This is the medical term used when the blood becomes more acidic than it should be. Acidosis is common in cats with urethral obstruction since urine excretion is required to maintain normal blood acid levels. Affected cats can feel very unwell and if severe enough, acidosis can be fatal. Treatment with intravenous fluids in combination with relieving the urethral obstruction is often effective in correcting the acidosis. In very severe cases, other treatments such as sodium bicarbonate may be required

- Azotaemia and acute kidney injury (AKI): Failure of urine excretion due to urethral obstruction or rupture of the bladder can cause AKI. AKI is diagnosed by measuring blood levels of urea and creatinine – two waste products that are normally excreted by the kidneys. The AKI is generally fully reversible if treated promptly by relieving the obstruction/repairing the bladder rupture, giving intravenous fluids and correcting any complications that might be present such as dehydration and hyperkalaemia

- Dehydration: vomiting in addition to not eating or drinking can quickly cause dehydration and if left untreated this can be fatal. Treatment involves intravenous fluids – placing your cat on a drip

Treatment of the obstruction generally requires sedation or anaesthesia. Pain relieving treatment – analgesia – is also required. Many vets prefer anaesthesia as this ensures that the urethra is as relaxed as possible and the cat is completely unaware of what is happening. Where possible, the obstruction is relieved by passing a soft, lubricated tube (a urinary catheter) into the bladder. The bladder may need to be emptied by cystocentesis first in severe cases. The urethra may need to be flushed with saline (salt) solution to clear blockages caused by small stones or urine-sand (debris such as crystals from the urine which have compacted to a sandy sludge). Massage of the urethra using a finger in the cat's rectum can help to dislodge obstructions and allow these to be flushed back to the bladder. Repeat filling and drainage of the bladder with saline solution also helps to remove blood clots, urine-sand and very small stones. The bladder is then emptied and the urinary catheter is usually left in for between 1 and 4 days to allow any urethral trauma to heal. Depending on their type, any stones flushed back to the bladder can be removed by bladder surgery or dissolved by feeding a special diet.

In some cases, a urinary catheter cannot be passed along the urethra. In these cases, surgical procedures can be done to allow urine in the bladder to empty via a plastic tube to the outside (e.g. tube cystotomy or tube urethrostomy). This is often a useful temporary procedure while the urethral disease is treated. In cases where the urethral disease cannot be treated, a permanent urethrostomy, re-plumbing the urethra, can be done.

SECTION 2 | explaining the science of lower urinary tract disease

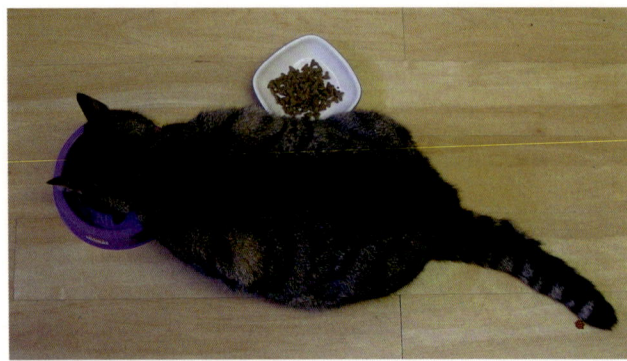

A number of prescription diets have been designed to help cats with FLUTD.

2. Treatment of cats with urethral plugs

Urethral plugs are made of a protein matrix which can also have trapped crystals in it. The plugs are a cause of urethral obstruction so initial treatment is as discussed above.

In the long-term, cats that have had urethral plugs may also need the following:

- Treatments aimed at reducing the numbers of crystals in the urine. Although it is normal for cats to produce crystals in their urine, especially if they are fed a standard dry diet, reduction of crystal numbers can help to reduce the formation of plugs. Measures which encourage production of more dilute urine are also helpful. For example, feeding a diet specifically formulated to encourage drinking by stimulating your cat's sensation of thirst may be helpful. These diets are available in both dry and wet form. Your cat should also be encouraged to drink more using the tactics discussed in the section Treatment of cats with FIC

- Treatment aimed at reducing urethral spasm. Some cats benefit from treatment with drugs that relax the muscle around the urethra such as those discussed in the section Treatment of cats with urethral spasm

- Treatments such as those discussed in the FIC treatment section. These help to reduce inflammation of the bladder and therefore reduce production of the protein matrix. Production of more dilute urine also helps to reduce the likelihood of plugs forming

3. Treatment of cats with uroliths

The most common type of urinary stones are calcium oxalate and struvite. Stones can be located at various sites in the urinary tract including the kidneys (nephroliths), ureter (ureteroliths), bladder (cystic calculi) and urethra. The bladder and the urethra are the most common location for stones. The clinical signs vary according to the site of the stone – for example typical signs of FLUTD are seen with bladder stones. Stones are diagnosed in a variety of ways:

- Radiography (x-rays) can be helpful in visualising stones. Unfortunately not all stones are radiodense (show up on a standard 'plain' x-ray) although contrast studies can help to find these

- Ultrasound is very helpful in imaging stones and is a very non-invasive test that can usually be performed without sedation or anaesthesia. Unfortunately ultrasound cannot examine the whole of the urinary tract – for example it is not possible to image all of the urethra using this technique so stones in this location may be missed

SECTION 2 | explaining the science of lower urinary tract disease

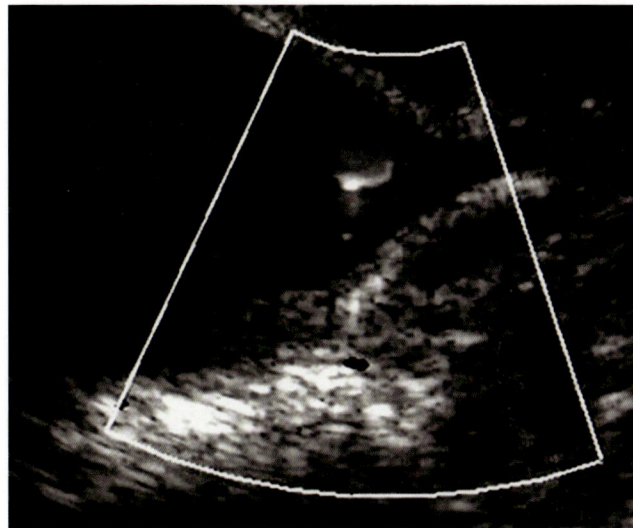

This ultrasound picture of a bladder shows a small stone. The area of interest is outlined by a white line. Urine in the bladder is black, the bladder wall is white and the stone is circular and bright white.

- Very small stones may be seen in a free-catch or catheter urine sample

- Urinalysis can give some clues as to the type of bladder stone – for example if crystals are present they are usually the same type as the stone. Unfortunately this is not consistently helpful – not all cats with stones will have crystals in their urine and in a small number of cases, the crystals will be different in type to the stone

- Precise diagnosis of the stone type requires specialist analysis of the stone itself and this procedure usually takes a few weeks to perform

In cats suffering from urolithiasis for the first time, many vets recommend surgical removal to ensure that the stone is typed and the correct longterm treatment is prescribed.

Struvite stones can be treated very effectively using special prescription diets. The struvite stones are dissolved in the bladder over a period of a few weeks. Use of struvite dissolution diets is not appropriate for all cats, however, so it is important to follow your veterinarian's advice, not only on the type of diet, but also the feeding duration. For example, struvite dissolution diets are generally not used for more than two months.

Urethral struvite stones can be flushed back into the bladder for dissolution (by a procedure known as 'retrograde hydropulsion') or expelled from the body by a procedure called 'voiding hydropulsion'. Both of these procedures require anaesthesia and often need a specialist to perform them.

Oxalate stones cannot be treated medically – there are no diets that can cause these stones to dissolve. Therefore oxalate stones need to be removed surgically. Urethral oxalate stones can be flushed back to the bladder for surgical removal from here or they can be expelled from the body using voiding hydropulsion.

Kidney stones are harder to treat and it is often better to leave these alone unless they are causing specific problems – for example obstructing flow of urine from the kidney into the ureter. Cats with kidney stones may be more vulnerable to bacterial infections and therefore may need long courses of antibiotics.

Ureteral stones (stones in the ureter) can also be hard to treat. In some cases, certain drugs can help to relax the muscle of the ureter and so enable passage of the stone/s into the bladder.

SECTION 2 | explaining the science of lower urinary tract disease

> **Use a glass, metal or ceramic water bowl and fill it to the brim to encourage your cat to drink more.**

Lithotripsy is a newer procedure using mechanical techniques and/or shock waves to break up stones into pieces small enough to be passed with the urine, or be passed from the kidney to the bladder for removal at surgery. This is a procedure which is only available in a small number of specialist clinics at the moment and has been mainly used to treat stones in the kidneys and ureters of dogs.

Prevention of urolithiasis

Cats that have suffered from urinary stones are vulnerable to repeat episodes of this problem. Fortunately, several diets are available that help reduce the risk of recurrence of stones. However, the type of diet will depend on the type of stone your cat suffered from and their other medical and lifestyle requirements.

Important factors in maintaining good urinary tract health and helping to prevent FLUTD include:

- Where possible feed a moist diet (cans or pouches) or a diet designed to promote urine dilution. Producing a urine with a specific gravity less than 1.035 helps to reduce the formation of stones by being more dilute and encouraging the cat to urinate more frequently

- Encourage the cat to drink as much as possible (discussed later in the section on Treatment of FIC)

Prescription diets often have other modifications including supplemental omega 3 and 6 fatty acids for an anti-inflammatory effect, or additional anti-oxidants.

4. Treatment of cats with urethral spasm

Urethral spasm is the medical term for an involuntary tightening of the muscles around the urethra and can occur with any of the causes of lower urinary tract disease in cats. Spasm is painful and can cause urethral obstruction by preventing the passage of urine. The urethral wall has two types of muscle in it – smooth muscle and skeletal (also known as striated) muscle. A variety of drugs can be given to treat spasm and your veterinarian will base their choice on the individual needs of your cat.

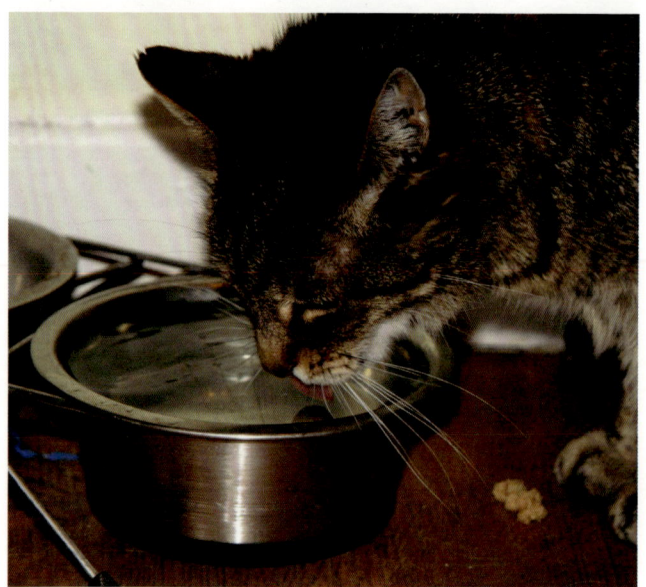

Encouraging your cat to drink more water helps to prevent future episodes of FLUTD.

SECTION 2 | explaining the science of lower urinary tract disease

5. Treatment of cats with bladder diverticula
A bladder diverticulum is a small outpouching of bladder lining through the bladder wall and can be seen as a congenital defect or in association with FLUTD. In cats with FLUTD, the diverticulum may spontaneously disappear once the cause of the FLUTD is treated. If the diverticulum remains then surgical removal might be advised. If this is done then it is normal for the removed portion of bladder to be submitted for histopathology (analysis by a pathologist) and bacterial culture (to check for bacterial infection of the tissue).

6. Treatment of cats with bladder tumours
Where possible, the recommended treatment for bladder tumours is surgical removal. Unfortunately, since cats are very good at hiding disease the disease is often very advanced by the time many of these cancers are diagnosed. It may not be possible to remove the cancer in the following situations:

- The cancer is so advanced that too little healthy bladder tissue remains to function. In some specialist institutions, procedures using bowel tissue as a graft can be done. This procedure replaces the cancerous tissue with healthy bowel tissue
- The diseased portion of the bladder involves the bladder neck or other vital structures such as the ureters. Tumours in the bladder neck (also referred to as the 'trigone') are difficult or impossible to remove since all of the vital structures (such as the ureters and the urethra) enter and exit the bladder in this area
- The cancer has already spread elsewhere in which case surgery to remove the primary (original) lesion is pointless. The most common location for bladder cancer to spread to is the lungs. This is one reason why a chest x-ray may be performed in your cat when a tumour is found
- The cat is suffering from significant other problems which make anaesthesia or surgery hazardous. For example, in a cat that also has severe kidney disease, anaesthesia risks precipitation of a crisis

In those cats where surgery cannot be done and in those where it has not been possible to completely remove the cancer, palliative treatment might be recommended. This involves therapy to improve the quality of life such as painkillers. As always, your vet is the best person to advise you on the use of these drugs.

7. Treatment of cats with bacterial urinary tract infections
If your cat has been diagnosed with a bacterial urinary tract infection then a course of antibiotics will be recommended. The type of antibiotic and length of course depends on factors including the type of infection, whether or not there are any other problems such as bladder stones which also need to be treated and results of the bacterial culture and sensitivity test. The sensitivity test evaluates the ability of several different antibiotics to slow or stop the growth of the bacteria in laboratory conditions.

Where concurrent kidney disease is also present, it is not unusual to prescribe a six week course of antibiotics.

Recurrent infections need repeat courses of treatment so your vet may recommend that repeat bacterial cultures are performed on urine samples periodically to monitor progress. Unfortunately antibiotic resistance can occur necessitating a change in the type of antibiotic prescribed.

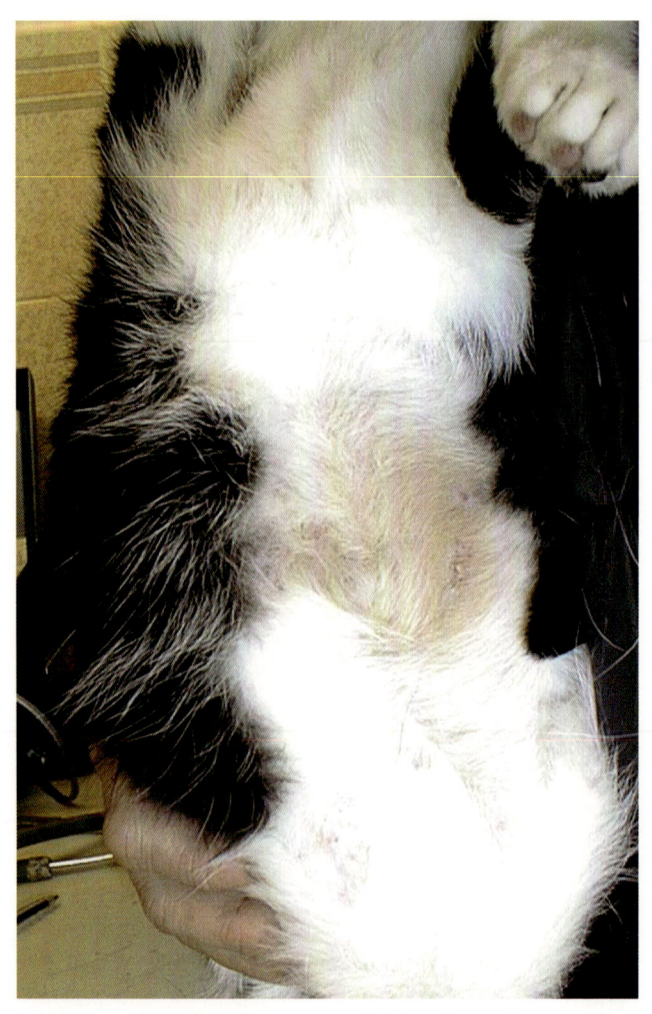

SECTION 2 | explaining the science of lower urinary tract disease

Over-grooming the belly (left) or perineum (right) can be seen in some cats with FLUTD.

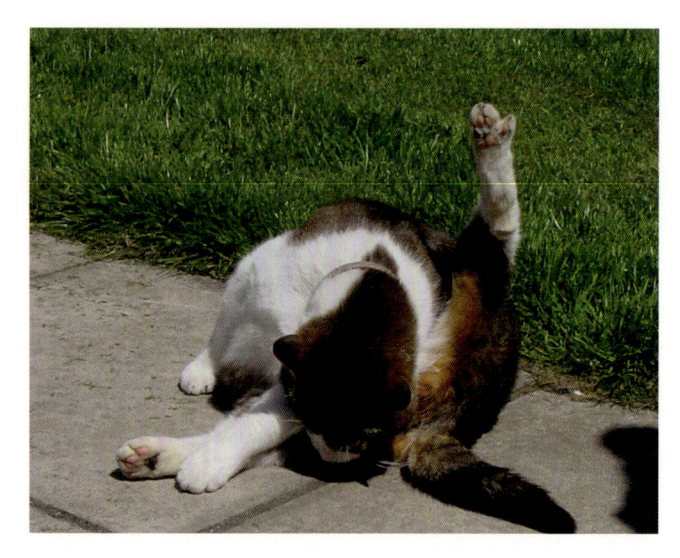

8. Treatment of cats with FIC

Non-obstructive FIC is considered to be a self-limiting problem – in other words cats get better without any treatment. For several good reasons, treatment is recommended in spite of this:

- Recovery from FIC can take up to 10 days
- FIC can be a very painful and distressing condition
- Cats with FIC may self-traumatise their perineum (the area around the anus, vulva or penis) in response to the pain
- Cats with FIC may stop eating in response to the pain. If a cat doesn't eat for three days or longer there is a risk of them developing a potentially fatal illness called hepatic lipidosis (where fat accumulates in their liver). This risk is higher in overweight cats, as are many cats with FIC

SECTION 2 | explaining the science of lower urinary tract disease

- Male cats with FIC are vulnerable to developing urethral obstruction which, if not treated rapidly, can be fatal
- Cats with FIC can develop behavioural problems such as:
  - Over-grooming their belly or perineum. This can be severe enough to make these areas bald
  - Becoming more aggressive to their owner and other animals in the house
  - Inappropriate urination, for example urinating inside the house and not in a litter box
- Having a cat with FIC is often very distressing to the owner

Although FIC is common and has been a subject of much research, very few treatments have been assessed in a rigorous way. For example, not all of the treatment trials have included a 'placebo' (control) group. So-called 'un-controlled' studies are very vulnerable to showing misleading results since owners and vets are always keen for a new treatment to be effective and it's easy for this enthusiasm to bias results. FIC usually resolves spontaneously, often within a few days, so many treatments can appear to be effective when in fact the cat is making a spontaneous recovery.

All of the current medical treatments for FIC are palliative – in other words only aiming to support the cat through an episode and reduce the risk of further episodes from occurring. The biggest long-term improvements are seen using a dual approach to reduce stress and encourage the cat to produce dilute urine.

1. Strategies to reduce stress in the home.
Since stress is known to play a critical role in causing FIC, it follows that reducing stress is highly desirable. Known stressors include:

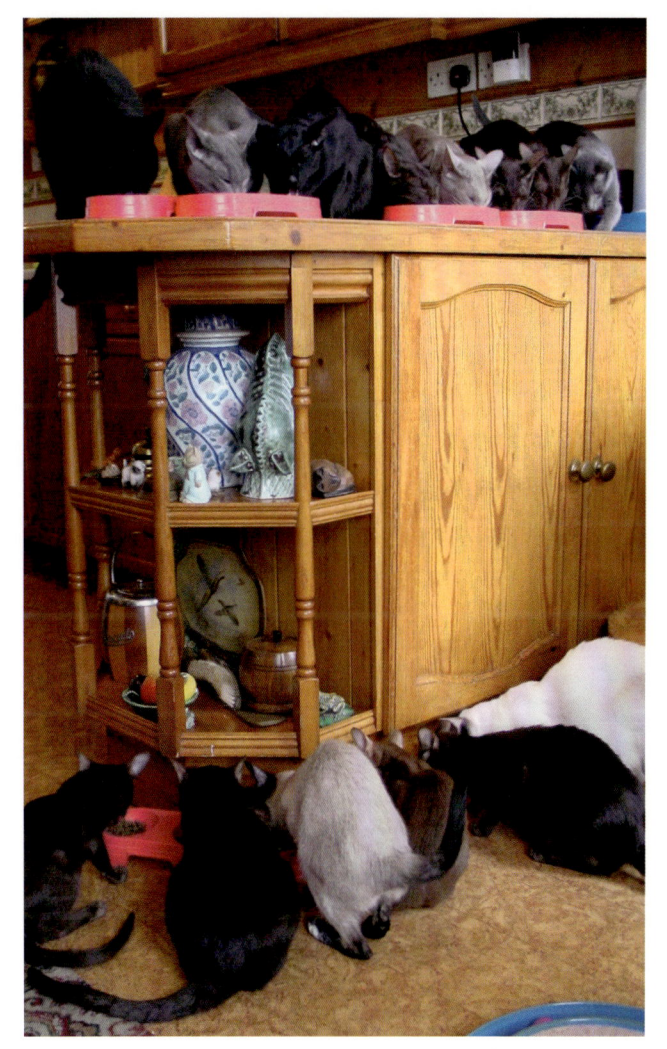

Cats from different social groups should not be expected to come together to feed as this can be very stressful. Ideally all cats should be able to eat alone.

SECTION 2 | explaining the science of lower urinary tract disease

- Living with another cat with which the FIC cat is in conflict (in other words, cats belonging to different social groups). Stress or conflict with other cats in the neighbourhood can also be a factor and should be considered for cats in single cat households
- Sudden changes to the diet
- Sudden changes in the environment – for example building work in the home, moving house and so on
- Sudden changes in the weather which might affect a cats' desire to go outdoors
- Addition of new pets or people into the household

Useful strategies might include:

- Reading literature on the Indoor Cat Initiative – a superb website devoted to providing information to enrich the lives of indoor cats: http://indoorpet.osu.edu The website is full of information on normal feline behaviour and feline needs in a very readable form
- Consulting a veterinary behaviourist or other suitably qualified behavioural expert to discuss what stressors may be present in your household and how you can address these. Your veterinary surgeon will be able to refer you to someone with appropriate qualifications
- If referral to a behavioural expert is not possible then factors you should look at yourself include:

i) Where are the litter boxes sited in the home?

Consider moving these if they are in busy areas where the cat might feel anxious when using them.

Assess whether there is any possibility of a cat from another household being able to see the FIC cat when it is using the litter box – for example through windows. Assess the area as if you are a cat to see where these observation points might exist. If this is a possibility then it's worthwhile considering:

– Investing in semi-opaque coverings for windows so a cat can't see in

– Reducing the availability of resting places where other cats can sit and watch your cat – for example by moving plant pots to stop a cat sitting in a certain place

– Blocking the line of view another cat might have by moving garden furniture and plants pots

ii) Consider investing in a secure cat-flap which only opens when cats with the correct microchips attempt to use it.

iii) Consider the availability of resources within the home. The five essential resources a cat needs are food, water, litter boxes, resting areas and points of entry and exit into the territory. Cats are by nature solitary hunters and have a low requirement for social interaction. They naturally live in groups of related individuals and are hostile to intrusion by cats from other social groups. Even in multi-cat households, several social groups may exist and each of these groups needs its own separate resources – they will not enjoy having to share resources. Therefore the distribution of resources in the home is a key factor in minimising stress.

Step 1: identify the number of social groups there are in your house. It is not always obvious how many social groups exist within one household. It is helpful to make a record of tactile

SECTION 2 | explaining the science of lower urinary tract disease

> **The five essential resources a cat needs are food, water, litter boxes, resting areas and points of entry and exit into the territory.**

behaviour shown between cats – examples include rubbing and grooming. Cats in the same social groups tend to rub and groom one another while cats in separate social groups do not. If you write the names of all of your cats on a piece of paper and then draw arrows between the names whenever you see them either rub or groom each other you will build up a picture which helps you to identify the social groups. Some cats can be in more than one group so it can get a little complicated. Once you know how many groups of cats you have in your household you can then start to ensure that resources are distributed appropriately in the house so that each cat can gain free and immediate access to all resources at all times, without running the gauntlet of cats from other social groups.

Step 2: consider the food supply in the home. Cats prefer to eat on their own. Ideally food should be offered on an ad lib basis and if kittens are fed in this way from weaning onwards they will usually successfully control their food intake. However changing to an ad lib system when cats have already been used to a meal feeding system can be associated with problems of over eating and therefore you need to discuss this issue with your veterinary surgeon before making any changes. In multi-cat households, it is essential to have several 'feeding stations'. Cats from different social groups should not be expected to come together to feed as this is very stressful; ideally all cats should be able to eat alone.

Step 3: consider the water supply in the home. Cats prefer to eat and drink in different places in the house so water and food bowls should not be placed next to each other and use of double bowls with food on one side and water on the other is not advised. Cats will not voluntarily drink as much if their water bowl is by their food bowl. Separate drinking facilities should be provided for each of the social groups in the household. Other factors which can help to encourage drinking include:

– Type of water bowl: cats usually prefer to drink from metal, glass or ceramic bowls rather than plastic ones

– Size of water bowl: the bowl should have a large diameter – cats do not usually like their whiskers to touch the side of their food or water bowl. A large bowl also ensures a large surface area for drinking. Cats do not usually like to place their heads directly over the bowl or into it to drink

– Amount of water: the bowl should be filled to the brim. Cats rarely drink from bowls that are not completely full as this requires them to put their head into the bowl

– Moving water: many cats like drinking moving water so providing a pet fountain can be helpful

– Experimenting with different types of water can be helpful – e.g. tap water, collected rain water and mineral water to see if your cat prefers water from different sources. You can

SECTION 2 | explaining the science of lower urinary tract disease

also consider flavouring the water but many cats will be less likely to drink if the water is significantly different from what they are used to and there are some flavourings that are toxic to cats (see section Helping your cat to produce dilute urine for more information on this)

Step 4: consider the supply of litter boxes in the home. Stress associated with urination can be a significant factor in FIC cases. The ideal litter box is safe, secure and private with no conflict associated with using this area of the home (or outside if this is where the cat urinates). In multi-cat households there should be sufficient litter boxes to cater to all of the social groups and these should be positioned in such a way that the cat does not have to pass cats from other social groups to access the litter box. The number of litter boxes should correlate with the number of social groups in the household. Covered litter boxes can be unpopular with some cats as they can leave cats vulnerable to an ambush by another cat. Litter box hygiene is essential so that there is nothing to put a cat off toileting in the box. Daily scooping of urine and faeces is essential and full cleaning of the box with replacement of the litter should take place at least once a week. The litter type should be selected to be one which the cat likes to use – perfumed or uncomfortable litters (e.g. some cats dislike different consistencies of litter) should be avoided. The depth of the litter has been shown to be important in encouraging appropriate toileting behaviour – where possible deep litter boxes should be used and filled so that the cat can dig and bury its urine and faeces deposits adequately. In older cats, deep litter boxes can be difficult to climb into so a ramp might be needed. Alternatively, a tray with a shallow entrance (like a potting tray) can be used, or you can cut a shallow-sided entrance into a normal litter box.

Step 5: consider the supply of resting areas in the home. When in situations of tension, a cat will try to escape to a safe location. It is therefore important to provide sufficient resting places, including some at elevated locations (for example on top of a cupboard) since cats feel safer in higher places. There should be plenty of opportunities for the cat to hide and have privacy – for example providing cardboard boxes with blankets can be very helpful.

Step 6: consider the entry and exit points in the home. Conflict associated with entry or exit of the territory can be a significant source of stress. It is therefore important to try and

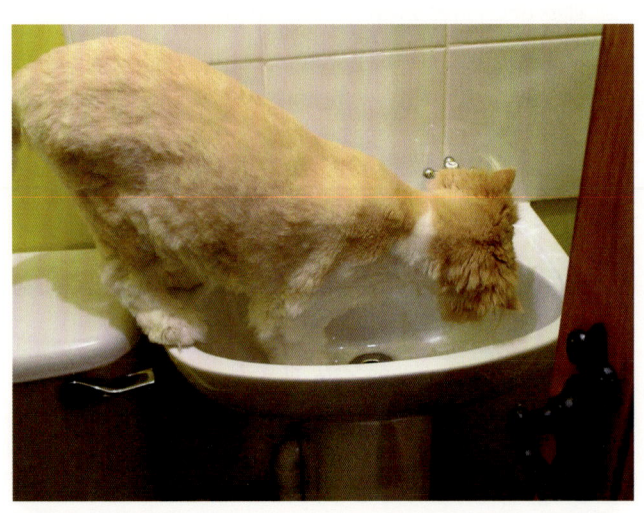

Some cats like drinking from moving water sources such as pet fountains and dripping taps.

SECTION 2 | explaining the science of lower urinary tract disease

facilitate separate entry and exit points so that each cat can come into or leave the home (or area of potential conflict) without running the gauntlet of other individuals.

- Use of feline pheromones: pheromones are chemicals which cats use to communicate with each other. For example, when your cat rubs their head on your legs they are transferring pheromones which signify that you are a friend and not something to fear. Synthetic preparations of feline facial pheromone complex F3 are available commercially. F3 is also known as the 'familiarisation pheromone' since it decreases the perception of threat and increases a feeling of safety in the home. Synthetic preparations of F3 pheromone may be helpful in reducing tension found in multicat households. F3 acts as a confirmatory signal that the environment is safe and therefore should be used in conjunction with other environmental management, such as ensuring that there are adequate litter boxes and so on. Used alone, synthetic preparations of F3 pheromone are not sufficient to prevent signs of FIC associated with stress but they can be very helpful if introduced just prior to periods of increased stress – for example if a new cat is to be introduced to the house. The pheromone product should be used for at least a month, starting a few days before the arrival of the new cat and the period of use may be extended in accordance with advice from a veterinarian or behaviourist

When in situations of tension, a cat will try to escape to a safe location.

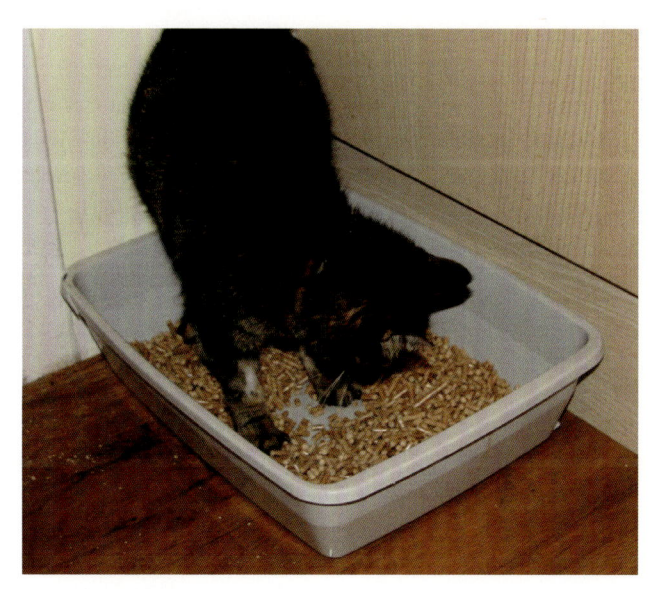

Litter trays should always be clean and situated in quiet areas where the cat can have some privacy.

- Environmental enrichment as a way of reducing stress. Examples of positive ways of improving a cat's environment include provision of climbing frames with resting areas and playing games that stimulate natural cat behaviour. For example providing paper bags and boxes for the cat to play in, fishing rod toys to chase and hunting games (e.g. hide toys filled with catnip or small pieces of food)

- Managing social stress: restricting (or reducing) the number of cats in the home to socially compatible levels and resisting the temptation to expand the household by introducing new

SECTION 2 | explaining the science of lower urinary tract disease

cats will help to reduce the incidence of stress-related diseases like FIC. FIC is very common in households where there are large numbers of cats

- Use of medication to reduce stress: although all of the above measures are essential in reducing stress in the home, in some cases additional therapy may be needed, at least for a while. Nutritional supplements or over the counter medications may be helpful in some cases, while other cats may need prescription medication. In all cases, veterinary advice is indispensible

2. Help your cat to produce dilute urine.
It is currently believed that the single most important dietary manipulation which helps to reduce the frequency and severity of FIC episodes is the rate of water turnover. In other words, your cat will be less likely to suffer from episodes of FIC if they produce dilute urine. Dilute urine is less painful to a diseased bladder so this will help to reduce the bladder pain associated with FIC. Producing more dilute urine does not treat the underlying cause of FIC so issues such as stress, discussed above, also need to be addressed. The aim is for your cat to be producing urine with a specific gravity around 1.035. This encourages frequent urination and dilutes any irritant components of the urine. Strategies to encourage production of dilute urine include:

- Ensure that you have followed the advice regarding the location, type of water bowl and so on, as discussed above

- Feed a wet rather than dry diet. If your cat will not eat a wet diet, then it is worth adding water to their cat biscuits and seeing if they will eat this. A good way of doing this is to gradually increase the amount of water added. Adding water to wet food can also help to increase fluid intake and hence encourage production of dilute urine. Some cats will tolerate a food that resembles soup!

- Feeding a diet specifically formulated to encourage drinking by stimulating your cat's sensation of thirst may also be helpful. These diets are available in both dry and wet form

- Ensure that water supplies are always easily accessible to your cat – for example on every floor of the house and never too far away from where your cat may be sitting or sleeping. Also ensure that access to water is not being restricted by social tensions in the home. For example, ensure that there is at least one water station per social group of cats in the household

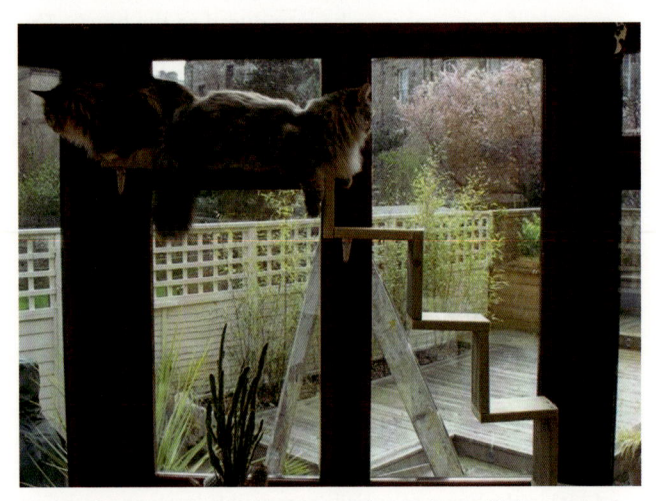

Climbing frames, interesting views from windows and toys all help to make the life of an indoor-only cat as stimulating as possible.

SECTION 2 | explaining the science of lower urinary tract disease

> Adding water to wet food can help to increase fluid intake and hence encourage production of dilute urine.

Offering flavoured water may encourage your cat to drink more but it must not be a salty liquid as this can increase the risk of problems including high blood salt levels (hypernatraemia) and systemic hypertension (high blood pressure). Examples of ways to do this include:

- Poaching chicken or fish in unsalted water and offering the liquid to your cat as a drink (this can also be frozen and therefore used over a period of time)

- Offering juice from a drained can of tuna or salmon in spring water (not brine as this is very salty)

- Offering the liquid left when a bag of frozen cooked prawns is defrosted

- Liquidising fish or prawns in water to create a fishy broth. Again this can be frozen for future use. Some owners find freezing the liquid in ice cube trays helpful. A cube of frozen broth added to a bowl of water may be enough to stimulate drinking

- Water flavourers are available in some countries and may help cats to drink more. Do not use stock cubes as many of these contain onion powder which is poisonous to cats

- If you are unsure as to the safety of what you are thinking of offering your cat then discuss this with your veterinary surgeon

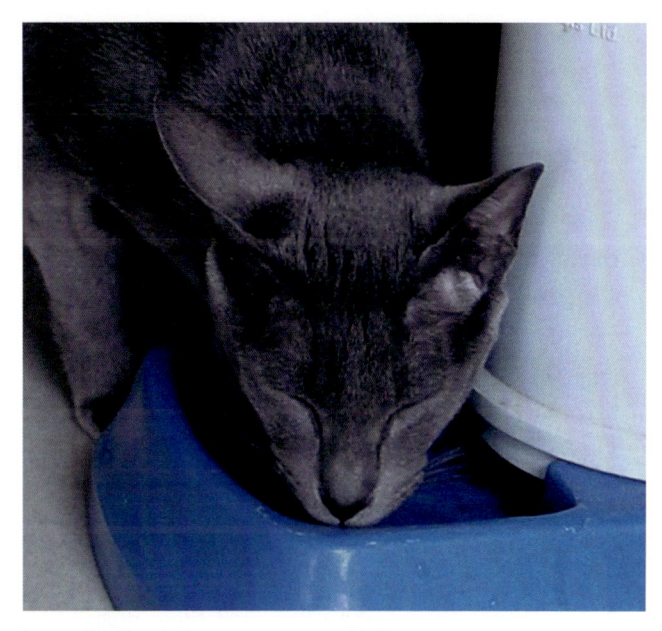

Ensure that there is always easy access to drinking water.

3. Medical treatments

A number of medical treatments may be suggested in cats with FIC. These include:

■ Painkillers and anti-inflammatory drugs: while painkillers have not been shown to alter the course of FIC, they can help an affected cat to feel as comfortable as possible. Examples include non steroidal anti-inflammatory agents and opiates. Glucocorticoid steroid drugs have been shown to be ineffective in treating FIC

SECTION 2 | explaining the science of lower urinary tract disease

- Therapy for urethral spasm as discussed earlier may be recommended in some cats with FIC

- Glycosaminoglycan (GAG) supplements. This is usually an oral treatment which is given with the aim of supplementing the GAG lining of the bladder and hence reduce the permeability of the bladder to noxious substances. Unfortunately, several clinical trials have shown that GAG supplements are not effective in the majority of cats affected by FIC

- Tricyclic antidepressants (TCAs) and Selective Serotonin reuptake inhibitors (SSRIs): These two groups of drugs have been found to be helpful in some people with interstitial cystitis and hence have also been trialled in cats with FIC. TCAs work by improving bladder capacity (allowing the bladder to fill with more urine) and have anti-inflammatory, pain-relieving and anti-depressant effects. Clinical trials have shown that short-term therapy (treatment for around 7 days) is not helpful and when used these drugs need to be administered for a period of three to six months. Unfortunately, well designed trials have not been done to assess the usefulness of this therapy over longer periods although many clinicians feel that TCAs can help some cats with FIC. TCAs can be associated with significant side-effects such as liver damage, sleepiness and urinary retention (accumulation of urine in the bladder since the cat doesn't feel aware that their bladder is full) and so are best reserved for severe cases of FIC or where a particular unavoidable short-term stress such as moving home is anticipated

- Cats receiving multiple therapies can be difficult to medicate. Medicating with multiple drugs can be made easier by using empty gelatine capsules available from a vet or pharmacist

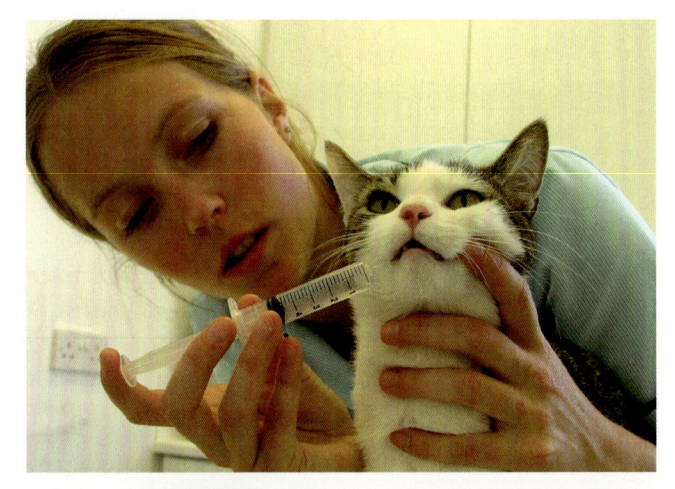

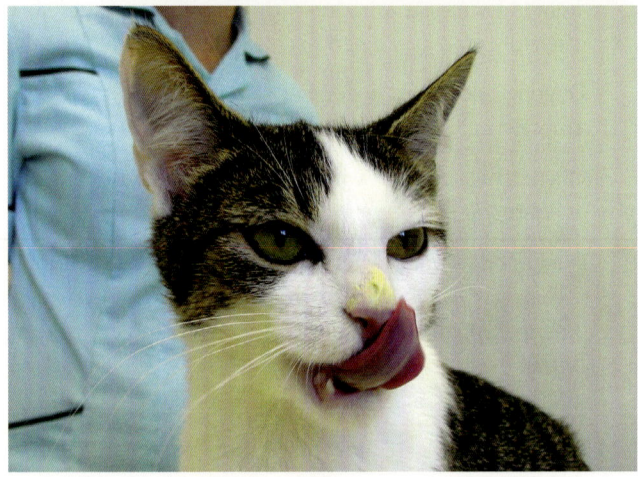

Syringing a small amount of water after giving a pill or capsule helps the medication to travel to the stomach quickly and without causing any irritation to the oesophagus (food pipe). Alternatively a small amount of butter can be put on the cat's nose – licking this off also helps any pills and capsules to travel quickly to the stomach.

SECTION 2 | explaining the science of lower urinary tract disease

The capsule is opened, the appropriate drugs are added and then the capsule is closed again. This means that it is possible to dose a cat with two or more medicines in one go – likely to be much more popular with the cat than giving multiple pills. Giving multiple medications can increase the risk of side-effects through drug interactions which is something for you and your vet to discuss and be aware of when working out a treatment regime for your cat. If you are finding it difficult to medicate your cat ask your vet to prioritise which treatments are most important so that you can ensure that your cat is getting the most important ones everyday

After any tablet or capsule medication is given the cat should be offered food or given a small amount of water to encourage the tablet to travel to the stomach. This is to prevent tablets or capsules from sitting in the food pipe (oesophagus) for prolonged periods where they can cause irritation and potentially serious and long-lasting problems such as strictures (narrowing of the food pipe).

The best outcome for a cat with FIC requires attention to all of the factors discussed in this section. Referral to a veterinary behavioural expert may be helpful in order to accurately diagnose and resolve causes of chronic stress in the home. In those cats that continue to suffer from episodic disease, owners can be helpful in detecting when an episode is about to occur (by recognising the so-called 'prodromal signs' that precede an episode). Examples of prodromal signs would include excessive licking of the perineum and changed behaviour such as being more irritable with other cats in the home. Action that might help to prevent an episode (or reduce its severity) include:

- Ensuring that synthetic F3 pheromone diffusers are renewed
- Using synthetic F3 pheromone spray in targeted areas like the cat's bed (not while he or she is in there!)
- Increasing fluid intake, using all of the strategies discussed earlier
- Considering an increase in therapy/ies shown to be helpful in previous episodes
- In some cats, extra attention in the form of TLC (tender loving care, cuddles etc) can help to prevent an episode from developing

This approach can also be helpful if a stressful event is anticipated (such as moving house) and thought to risk a recurrence of FIC.

What surgical treatment options are there?

In some cases, surgery is required to treat the cause of the FLUTD. Examples would include:

- Cystotomy: Opening the bladder up, for example to remove bladder stones which cannot be dissolved by a specifically formulated diet, or where the type of stone is not known
- Cystectomy: Surgery to remove part of the bladder – for example in a cat with a bladder tumour or bladder diverticulum
- Biopsy of the bladder wall or lesions via a cystotomy. This is indicated in some cats with thickened bladders or where there is a suspicion of cancer. The tissue removed is sent to a pathologist for special examination and so that a diagnosis can be made. In addition, bacterial culture of bladder tissue may be done to look for evidence of infection

SECTION 2 | explaining the science of lower urinary tract disease

> **The best outcome for a cat with FIC requires attention to all of the factors discussed in this section – especially addressing all of the possible causes of stress in the household.**

- Surgery to repair a ruptured (burst or leaking) bladder or urethra

- Tube cystotomy and urethrostomy: surgery to create a temporary connection between the bladder (cystotomy) or urethra (urethrostomy) and the outside. For example, in 'blocked' cats where it is not possible to pass a urinary catheter this can provide temporary relief while the urethral disease is treated

- Perineal urethrostomy: Surgery to create a new urethral opening following removal of the penis and final portion of urethra. This may be indicated in cats that have suffered from repeated urethral obstruction (for example if the cat has 'blocked' on 2 or more occasions in the past, your vet may suggest this treatment), cats with a urethral stricture or other causes of narrowing of the urethra. This treatment is only effective if the cause of the blockage is within the penis or very close to here

Side-effects are possible with all surgical procedures and your vet should discuss these with you before the surgery is performed. For example, cats that have had a large amount of their bladder removed may need to urinate several times an hour due to the small size of their bladder. Cats that have had a perineal urethrostomy are at an increased risk of urinary tract infections.

What is the prognosis (long-term outlook) for cats with FLUTD?

The long-term outlook for cats with FLUTD is very variable, depending on the cause of the disease. For example, cats with obstructive disease or bladder tumours have a poor prognosis. Around half of the cats diagnosed with urethral obstruction will continue to show signs of bladder discomfort, 30-40% will re-obstruct and 20% will be euthanased (put to sleep) because of continued disease.

In cats with non-obstructive FIC, there is no reduction in their expected lifespan, the main issue is the quality of their life. In some cats, the severity and frequency of episodes can be very distressing and if no treatment has been effective, euthanasia (putting your cat to sleep) may be the kindest option. Fortunately, many cats with FLUTD can be treated successfully and in those with FIC often the frequency and severity of episodes decreases with time. FIC is unusual in older cats since old age is often associated with a reduction in the urine concentration which is one of the treatments for FIC.

SECTION 3 | case illustration

Josh: a cat whose FLUTD is successfully managed by his owner

I got Josh and his brother Jess as kittens a short time after I lost my beloved dog, Lady. Both kittens were black, Jess short haired but Josh was long haired and fluffy. They came home with me and we went through all the usual kitten stuff, climbing walls and curtains etc, however, Josh was always closer to me and more dependant upon me than Jess.

When Josh was 2 years old he became ill and was 'blocked' due to FLUTD. He had a short stay at the vets and was unblocked and put on a special diet. This was difficult to administer with two cats as they both had to have the same diet which was expensive and Jess really did not like it. I told my vet my concerns and made the decision to keep both cats on wet food and leave cups of water in all areas of the house to encourage fluid intake. This worked for a while then Josh became ill again. After another few nights at the vets Josh came home and the vet asked me to monitor his progress for the weekend.

When I woke up on the Sunday morning Josh was sitting in the litter tray straining to pass urine. I was so upset and phoned the vet who told me that it sounded like Josh was 'blocked' again and put me in touch with the University for Small Animals in Edinburgh who said I should bring him in. On my way to the University I picked up my brother and we spoke about the probability that Josh might not pull through and if he did the financial implication of his treatment, which was an important consideration as I was on my own. My answer to this was if you have an animal you have to be prepared to do everything for them as a repayment for the love they give to you.

Josh and I were introduced to Danièlle Gunn-Moore at the University and the experience and knowledge she has with this debilitating – sometimes fatal – disease was like a breath of fresh air. Josh spent a long time in the hospital, however, I could go and visit him at night when I wanted. The support I was given was fantastic and every stage of Josh's progression was fully explained to me. Josh was found to have 'blocked' because of urethral spasm. When he recovered and came home Danièlle gave me tips on things that might cause Josh stress and could upset him again, things like changing furniture or surroundings that he was comfortable with. He came home with advice to continue feeding wet food and offering plenty of water as well as two different medications – one GAG supplement and a treatment for urethral spasm using a medicine which helped to relax the muscle of Josh's urethra making it easier for him to pass urine.

How do you cope with a cat with FLUTD that depends on constant medication?

I could set my clock by when Josh needs his tablet as he runs about the house meowing and jumps up on top of the work top where his tablet box sits. Getting a urine sample is equally easy. I totally empty and clean his litter tray then pop Josh in it. He seems to like peeing in an empty litter tray so all that is required is a syringe and sample bottle.

SECTION 3 | case illustration

Over a five to six year period Josh had medication comprising one daily tablet (GAG supplement) and an additional tablet every 8 hours (treatment for urethral spasm). Throughout this period we have had no mishaps and Josh has been contented and happy. Approximately one year ago Josh took a bad urine infection and had to go back up to the Hospital as an outpatient. Antibiotics soon cured this and the decision was taken to stop Josh's daily tablet and he has coped great on the 8 hourly tablets only.

I have also had invaluable support and expertise from Danièlle and her team. The things I have found hard to cope with are the stress of when he is ill and how useless I feel because I cannot take away the discomfort he is in. It is so heart breaking to see Josh straining to pass urine and when he gets relief it exhausts him so much he has to sleep for an hour or so, but I now know how to check his temperature by touching the inside of his ears and how they tend to get cooler after he has slept it off.

I have never regretted the decision I made the day I took Josh to the University Hospital. He still needs medication every 8 hours and things like nights out, holidays and even working flexible shifts are difficult to work in with Josh's tablet times but we get there. I met my partner four years ago and you maybe excused for thinking I am neurotic but my biggest concern when Keith and I decided to live together was how would Josh cope with another set of feet in the house or someone else other than him getting his "mum's" attention. Thankfully we are all coping well and Josh even lets Keith give him his tablet.

I consider myself to be very lucky as I still have Josh and have enjoyed many years with him. In comparison, my cousin has lost a cat to this disease and her new cat has also just been diagnosed with FLUTD. Josh is nearly 11 years old now but he is still fit for an old boy and can clean jump up from the floor to my full height (about 5 foot 4 inches) for a cuddle. All he asks for is a clean litter tray, his food twice daily and lots of cuddles – which he gets!

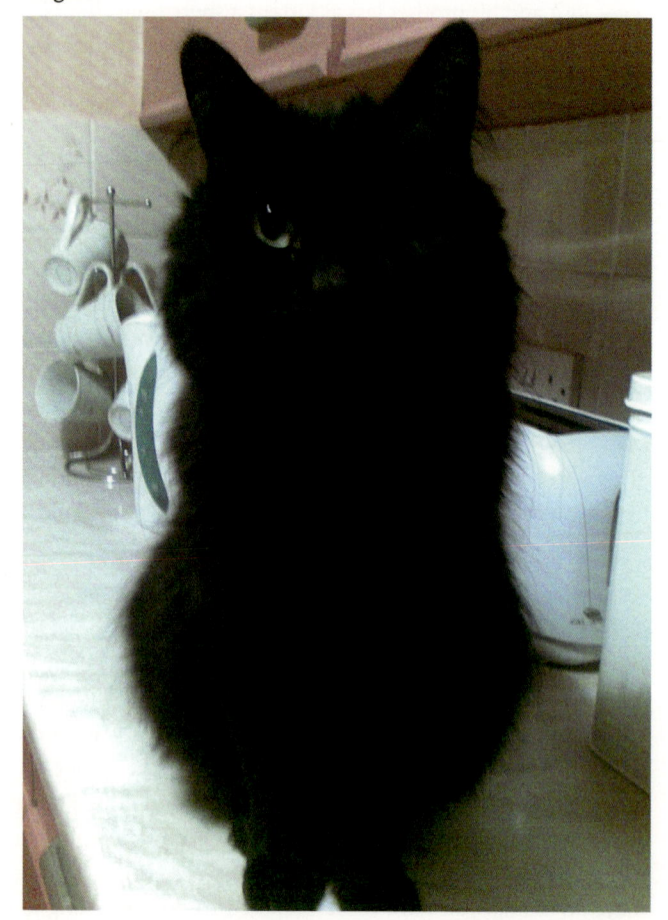

Josh waiting to get his tablet.

SECTION 4 | discussing your cat with your vet

A good relationship with your vet is vital to the care and wellbeing of your cat with FLUTD. It is important therefore that you feel able to discuss all of your concerns openly. Your vet is in the best position to advise you regarding specific questions on treatment and prognosis. You should feel able to ask your vet any questions and they should be able to explain things to you clearly in a way you can understand.

If you feel that the relationship you have with your vet is not answering your concerns then you can ask to see another vet within the practice, or look for another practice. Do not feel uncomfortable if you want to do this – your vet should not mind and it is within your rights to choose the vet you feel is best able to look after your cat. It is always worthwhile asking if there is anyone in the practice who is particularly interested in cat medicine. A number of feline-only practices also exist and you may be fortunate in finding one of these in your area.

Veterinary surgeons specialising in feline medicine can be contacted by your vet for further advice, if needed, or referral to a specialist can be arranged.

In order for your vet to be able to provide the level of care you are looking for with your cat, they will need to understand things from your perspective. For example:

- Will you be able to medicate your cat at home or is this out of the question (for example because your cat is very feisty or because you have severe arthritis in your fingers)? Will giving some medications be possible (e.g. dietary treatment) but others not possible (e.g. tablets)?

> **A good relationship with your vet is vital to the care and wellbeing of your cat with FLUTD. It is important therefore that you feel able to discuss all of your concerns openly.**

- What are your expectations for your cat? For example, would you prefer minimum intervention accepting a potentially shorter time with your cat or are you keen for your cat to have every possible treatment?

- Are finances limited in which case certain treatments may be too expensive? Your vet will be able to advise you on the likely cost of treating your cat

- Are there any particular treatments which you object to being used in your cat?

Once both of you know what your expectations are then it should be possible to jointly work out a treatment plan that is appropriate for your cat. It is important to remember that all treatment plans can be modified – at any time – and that anything you agree to can be changed, if needed, in the future.

SECTION 5 | further information

The information in this section is relevant to owners of cats suffering from severe disease such as cancer and urethral obstruction where decisions may need to be made regarding euthanasia.

Knowing when to say 'goodbye'

How long has my cat got before he/she dies or needs putting to sleep (euthanasia)?
This is an impossible question to answer as it varies enormously from cat to cat. Most cats can live a normal quality of life for some years after a diagnosis of FLUTD has been made. Sadly some die or need to be put to sleep (euthanased) soon after the diagnosis is made. This generally depends on the specific cause of the FLUTD and how treatable this is. Your vet is in the best position to advise on your own cat and its likely prognosis.

Will I know when it's time to say goodbye to my cat and let him/her go?
It is very rare for a sick cat to die painlessly in their sleep – much though most owners would wish this to happen. Death tends to be a slow and distressing process and it is far kinder to intervene and ask a vet to put your cat to sleep (euthanase it) when the time has come than let your cat suffer a prolonged and possibly painful death. Urethral obstruction is an exception in that it can cause a painful death over a period of hours to a few days. For many owners, the thought of having their cat put to sleep is painful and worrying. Most owners feel that their cat should be put to sleep once their quality of life has deteriorated and there is no veterinary treatment that can help to improve this. Your vet should be able to support and guide you in making this decision – if you are at all worried then consult them for advice.

Quality of life is not easy to judge but guidelines include:

Specific questions relating to the FLUTD, especially relevant to cats with FIC:
a) Is your cat having episodes infrequently (for example twice a year) and/or when present these resolve within a couple of days?

b) OR, is your cat suffering from frequent and distressing episodes of FLUTD lasting for several days at a time?

Specific questions relating to the FLUTD, especially cats that have suffered from urethral obstruction:
a) Is your cat always able to pass urine?

b) OR, is your cat suffering from repeated and distressing problems of urethral obstruction?

Specific questions relating to the FLUTD, especially cats that have suffered from urolithiasis:
a) Is your cat now free from stones?

b) OR, is your cat suffering from repeated stone formation despite all of your best efforts?

General questions which can be useful when assessing quality of life:
Behaviour:
a) Is your cat still behaving in its normal way – following its usual routines and activities (e.g. spending the same amount of time grooming)? Is your cat interacting with you as normal?

SECTION 5 | further information

b) OR, has your cat become withdrawn and quiet, not interested in going outside (if normally allowed out) or in interacting with you and other animals in the home?

Appetite:

a) Is your cat still interested in food?

b) OR, has their appetite disappeared and getting them to eat has become a struggle?

Toileting behaviour:

a) Is your cat still passing urine and faeces in the litter tray (or outside in the garden) as is normal for them?

b) OR, has your cat started to pass urine and faeces in other places (such as on their bed or on your carpets and flooring)?

Vocalisation:

a) Is your cat as chatty as normal?

b) OR, has there been a change in the amount of vocalisation (increase or decrease) or the sound that your cat makes when miaowing?

Pain or distress:

a) Does your cat seem happy and comfortable?

b) OR, have you seen any sign of pain or discomfort – for example signs of fear or aggression when being handled or sitting in the same place for hours with a glazed expression?

Signs of illness:

a) Is your cat free of signs of illness?

b) OR, is it suffering from signs of illness such as vomiting, weight loss or constipation?

If you answer b) to any of the above questions then you should consult your vet for advice on whether there are any treatments that can help your cat to regain its quality of life. If there are, you need to consider whether to give these treatments a try before making any final decisions. In some cases of non-obstructive FIC, re-homing can be a successful option that is worth considering. Cats that are bullied or unhappy in their current household may be free of stress and illness if re-homed. Trial re-homing sessions – for example a week or two at a friend or relative's house – can be useful.

What does euthanasia involve?

For most veterinary surgeons, euthanasia involves giving an overdose injection of a barbiturate anaesthetic agent intravenously, usually into a vein in the front leg. Once the injection is started, the cat will lose consciousness within a few seconds and the heart should stop within a few minutes. Occasionally, the veins of the front leg can be very fragile and difficult to access so alternative injection sites need to be used – these include the kidneys and the liver. In any case, the process should be quick and painless.

Although the majority of cats are put to sleep at a veterinary practice, most vets will be happy to come to an owner's home to do this, if desired.

SECTION 5 | further information

What happens to my cat's body after they die or are euthanased (put to sleep)?

In general the options will be:

- Burying your cat's body at home
- Asking your vet to arrange cremation of your cat's body. If desired, you can ask for an individual cremation to be performed and for the ashes to be returned to you

Your vet will be able to discuss these options with you. It is worthwhile considering how you would like your cat to be put to sleep (should the need arise) and what you would like to happen to their body while your cat is still well. This will save you the added distress of these decisions when your cat dies.

How to cope with losing your cat

Is there support available for me in my grief?
Losing a beloved cat is always going to be a traumatic and distressing experience and you are likely to go through several acknowledged stages of grief. These include denial, anger, guilt, hopelessness/depression and finally acceptance. Most people experience at least two of these stages. Carers of cats with terminal illnesses such as bladder tumours may start to go through this process as soon as the diagnosis is made. Where this is the case, a further stage of grief – 'bargaining' – may also be experienced where an owner is keen for their cat to live to a certain point (for example, please let them live through Christmas so we can have this time together).

Hopefully you will have friends and family that will be able to provide some support to you throughout this period. If you don't, then consider talking to the vets or nurses at your veterinary practice, your doctor or a priest – all of whom should be able to offer support. There may also be local support groups available – your veterinary practice should know about these.

What about my other cat/s – are they likely to grieve?
Yes, it is possible although many cats with FIC are 'loners' that will not be missed at all! As with people, cats can show grief at the loss of a companion. The behaviour of a cat following the loss of a house-mate is very variable and unpredictable. Some cats seem completely unaffected by the loss, some appear happier once they are on their own whilst others may show signs of grief such as sleeping less, not eating, appearing to look for their lost companion and vocalising more or losing all interest in life.

This process can affect cats (and other animals) for up to a year following their loss. In most cases, signs of grief will disappear within 6 months. You can help affected cats in the following ways:

- Keep routines in the home the same

> **It is worthwhile considering how you would like your cat to be put to sleep (should the need arise) and what you would like to happen to their body while your cat is still well.**

SECTION 5 | further information

- If your cat has lost its appetite then try hand-feeding food that has been slightly warmed (to just below body temperature). Consult your vet if your cat has not eaten for three or more days. A complete loss of appetite can cause a potentially fatal liver disease called hepatic lipidosis

- Provide social interaction for your cat by spending more time with them, grooming them, talking to them and playing with them. Try to keep the interaction low key and avoid intense handling and cuddling which could appear restrictive from a feline point of view

- Don't immediately get a new cat. Although some cats will crave the company of a new companion, the majority of cats will be more upset and distressed if a new cat is introduced too soon. Many cats prefer to be in single cat households and it is impossible to predict what they will feel about a newcomer. So, if your cat seems happy after the loss of a house-mate do not get another cat. If, on the other hand, you are keen to expand the home or feel that your cat is 'lonely' then it is advisable to wait for at least a couple of months before considering introducing a new cat. If a new cat does move in it will need to bring with it a new supply of resources (food, water, resting places and latrines) which are placed in separate locations in the household from those resources that are currently being used by the resident cat

More information on feline bereavement is available on the International Cat Care (ICC) website: www.icatcare.org/advice/cat-health/euthanasia-cats. ICC also has advice on introducing a new cat which could be helpful once a decision has been made to get another cat: www.icatcare.org/advice/getting-cat

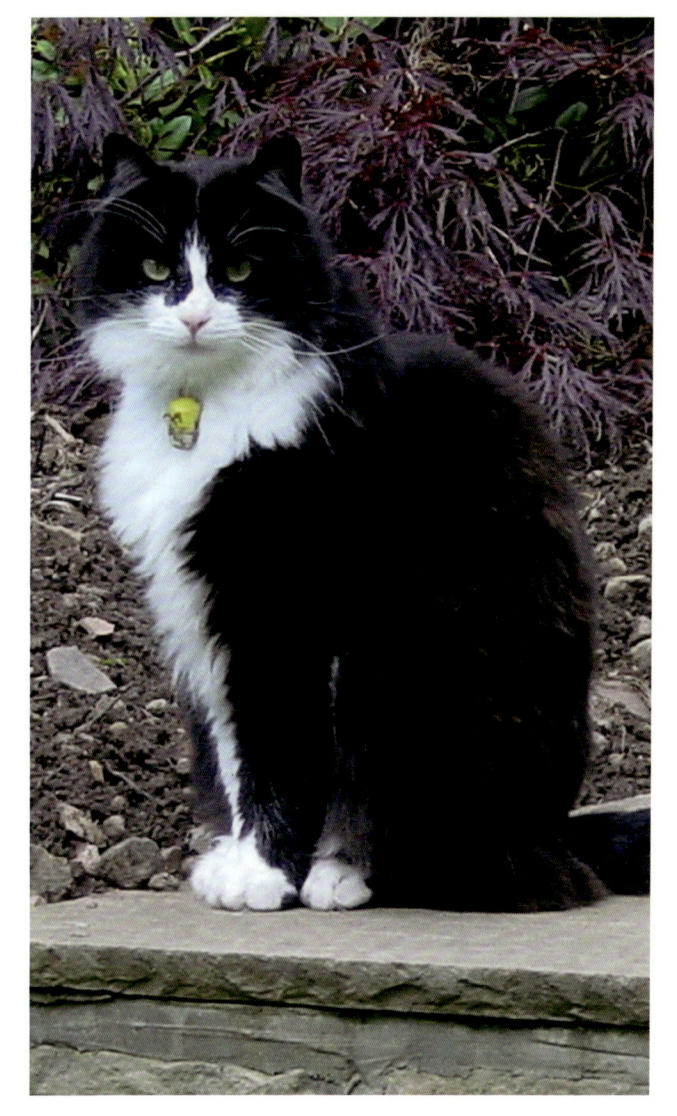

Useful websites and further reference sources

Several websites have been mentioned in this publication and you might find these interesting to look at:

General cat advice
International Cat Care: http://www.icatcare.org/

FLUTD information
ICC fact sheet on FLUTD http://www.icatcare.org/advice/feline-lower-urinary-tract-disease-flutd
ICC factsheet on spraying http://www.icatcare.org/advice/problem-behaviour/urine-spraying-cats

Feline behaviour and enriching your cat's life
The Indoor cat initiative http://indoorpet.osu.edu
ICC information on making your home 'cat friendly' http://www.icatcare.org/advice/keeping-your-cat-happy/making-your-home-cat-friendly

Bereavement support
http://www.icatcare.org/advice/cat-health/euthanasia-cats

Introducing a new cat to the home
http://www.icatcare.org/advice/getting-cat

Glossary of terms used by vets

Term	Definition
Acidosis	The blood is more acidic than normal. This is one potential consequence of urethral obstruction which can make affected cats lose their appetite, feel nauseous and generally unwell.
Acute kidney injury – AKI	Sudden loss of kidney function which can be caused by one or more of the following: ■ Reduced blood supply to the kidneys (so called pre-renal AKI). Causes include heart failure and dehydration. ■ Damage to the kidneys themselves (renal or intrinsic AKI). Causes include poisoning e.g. antifreeze (ethylene glycol), eating lilies. ■ Failure of urine excretion due to urethral obstruction or rupture of the bladder. This is called post-renal AKI. Although many causes of AKI are fully treatable (and the kidney damage can be reversed), if severe and untreated, AKI can progress to permanent chronic renal disease.
Anaesthesia	Providing a state of unconsciousness, muscle relaxation and loss of pain sensation using certain drugs (usually a combination of intravenously and by gas inhalation).
Azotaemia	Accumulation of protein breakdown products such as urea and creatinine in the blood. Measurement of urea and creatinine levels is used to diagnose kidney disease and dehydration. Cats with urethral obstruction often have an azotaemia since they cannot excrete their urine.
Biochemistry	Refers to blood tests of organ function (e.g. urea and creatinine), blood salt levels and protein levels.
Biopsy	Collection and laboratory analysis of a sample of tissue e.g. kidney biopsy.
Bladder	The bladder is a distensible, muscular sac where urine is stored. Urine is produced in the kidneys and passes to the bladder via the ureters. During urination, the bladder contracts and urine is passed through the urethra to the outside of the body.

Glossary of terms used by vets

Term	Definition
Bladder diverticulum	A bladder diverticulum is a small outpouching of bladder lining through the bladder wall and can be seen as a congenital defect or in association with FLUTD.
Clinical signs	The term used to describe what we would call our 'symptoms' if we were the cat e.g. sickness, loss of appetite.
Congenital	Congenital means present from birth.
Cystitis	Inflammation of the urinary bladder (where urine is stored before urination). One cause would be a bacterial infection of the urine.
Cystocentesis	Technique of urine collection using a needle and syringe. The needle is passed through the skin and into the bladder from which urine is collected.
Cystotomy	Surgery to open the bladder, for example to remove stones or place a temporary tube emptying urine from the bladder to the outside (tube cystotomy).
Dysuria	Showing pain and/or difficulty passing urine.
Euthanasia	Also referred to as 'putting to sleep' this is the term used when a vet ends a cat's life. This is usually done by giving an overdose of barbiturate anaesthetic into a vein – the cat dies within seconds of the injection being given.
Feline idiopathic cystitis (FIC)	Also known as idiopathic FLUTD (iFLUTD), this is the most common cause of FLUTD. Idiopathic means 'cause unknown' so this category is one where all of the known causes of FLUTD have been ruled out.
FLUTD	Feline lower urinary tract disease. FLUTD is the veterinary term used to describe a number of illnesses that can affect the bladder and/or urethra of cats.
Glycosaminoglycan (GAG)	A layer of glycosaminoglycans lines the internal surface of the bladder and is thought to help protect the bladder cells from noxious/irritating substances in the urine (such as acid, potassium, magnesium and calcium). The GAG layer also helps to stop bacteria and crystals in the urine from sticking to the bladder lining and causing problems.

Glossary of terms used by vets

Term	Definition
Haematology	Laboratory test assessing the blood count, numbers and types of white blood cells and platelets.
Haematuria	Passing red urine which may contain blood clots.
Histopathology	Microscopic examination of tissue samples by a pathologist. Histopathology is needed to make a diagnosis of, for example, cancer or inflammatory disease.
History taking	This is the process by which your vet gathers information on your cat and all of its problems (clinical signs).
Hyper-	Increased e.g. hyperkalaemia, hypercalcaemia: increased blood potassium levels, increased blood calcium levels.
Hypo-	Reduced e.g. hypokalaemia: low levels of potassium in the blood; hypotension: low blood pressure.
Idiopathic FLUTD	Spontaneous FLUTD where an underlying cause (such as infection or bladder stones) cannot be found.
Inflammation	A response of injured or damaged cells which helps to wall off the problem, eliminate infectious substances (for example) and restore healthy tissue. The classic signs of inflammation are: ■ Heat ■ Pain ■ Redness ■ Swelling ■ Loss of function.
Inflammatory	Pertaining to inflammation.
Kidney	Cats, like humans, have two kidneys located in their abdomen. The kidneys are bean shaped organs responsible for excreting waste products from the body in the form of urine.

Glossary of terms used by vets

Term	Definition
Non-obstructive FLUTD	This is the medical term used to describe FLUTD cases that are not suffering from urethral obstruction.
Obstructive FLUTD	This is the medical term used to describe FLUTD cases with urethral obstruction (ie 'blocked' cats).
Pathologist	A specialist in pathology who is able to diagnose the cause and/or type of disease by examining biopsy samples.
Pathology	The study of disease.
Perineum	The area adjacent to the anus and where the urethra exits.
Periuria	This is the medical term for urinating in inappropriate places rather than the litter box or garden. Common locations include carpet, duvets, sofas, baths and sinks.
Physical examination	Examination of body systems by a veterinary surgeon or nurse. Typically this includes listening to the chest, opening the mouth and feeling the tummy.
Pollakiuria	Increased frequency of urination.
Prognosis	A forecast of the likely long-term outlook for a cat with a given condition/s.
Pyelonephritis	Inflammation of the kidney often due to a bacterial infection.
Radiograph	X-ray.
Rectal examination	Insertion of a finger into the cat's rectum so that internal organs can be felt and assessed. For example the prostate gland can be felt using this test. This is a test which is usually done under deep sedation or anaesthesia.
Refractometer	An instrument that can measure the concentration of urine.
Sedation	Providing a state of calm and muscle relaxation using drugs. The cat is still conscious but, depending on the drugs used, may appear quite sleepy.

Glossary of terms used by vets

Term	Definition
Social groups	Cats living in groups tend to form relationships with other cats in the household. Like people, some cats get on better with each other than others. Cats in the same social group are happy to curl up together, rub and groom each th tother. If cats in the same home do not show this behaviour then they are likely to be in different social groups.
Spasm (urethral)	This is the medical term for an involuntary tightening of the muscles around the urethra and can occur with any of the causes of lower urinary tract disease in cats.
Spraying	Urine spraying is the term for depositing urine as a scent signal. To spray urine, the cat stands up, spraying a small amount of urine onto the vertical surface behind it. This differs from urination where the cat squats to pass urine onto a horizontal surface. Common locations for spraying include doors, windows, the area by the cat-flap and electrical equipment.
Stressor	An activity, event or other stimulus which causes stress in an individual. For example, moving house is considered to be stressful to cats as well as people.
Stricture	The medical term for an abnormal narrowing of a tube such as the urethra or the oesophagus (food pipe). Causes of strictures include tumours and inflammation.
Trauma	Injury or wound.
Ureter	Small tubes which take urine from each kidney to the bladder.
Urethra	The tube which carries urine from the bladder to the outside of the body.
Urethral obstruction	This is the medical term for a 'blocked' cat. A blockage in the urethra prevents the cat from being able to pass urine. This is an emergency condition since it can be fatal if left untreated.
Urethral plug	Urethral plugs are a potential cause of urethral obstruction which is a life-threatening condition. The plugs are made up of a protein matrix (a mixture of inflammatory proteins and mucus with cells and blood clots mixed in) often with some crystals (usually struvite).

Glossary of terms used by vets

Term	Definition
Urethrostomy	A connection from the urethra to the outside. In the case of a 'tube urethrostomy' this involves temporary placement of a tube which is removed once the urethra has healed. Permanent urethrostomies are done in some cases – for example perineal urethrostomy is helpful in cats that have a stricture in the penile urethra (urethra within their penis).
Urinalysis	Laboratory analysis of a urine sample e.g. concentration, number of cells, acidity, protein levels.
Urinary retention	Accumulation of urine in the bladder since the cat doesn't feel aware that their bladder is full.
Urolith, Urolithiasis	Urolithiasis is the medical term for stones (uroliths) which are most commonly located in the bladder (cystic uroliths).

Converting SI units to Conventional units and vice versa

Parameter	To convert Conventional to SI multiply by...	To convert SI to Conventional multiply by...
Urea	0.357	2.8
Creatinine	88.4	0.0113
Phosphate	0.323	3.1
Potassium	1	1
Sodium	1	1
Calcium	0.25	4
Albumin	10	0.1
Total protein	10	0.1
Bicarbonate	1	1
Packed cell volume (PCV) or haematocrit	0.01	100
Haemoglobin (Hb)	10	0.1

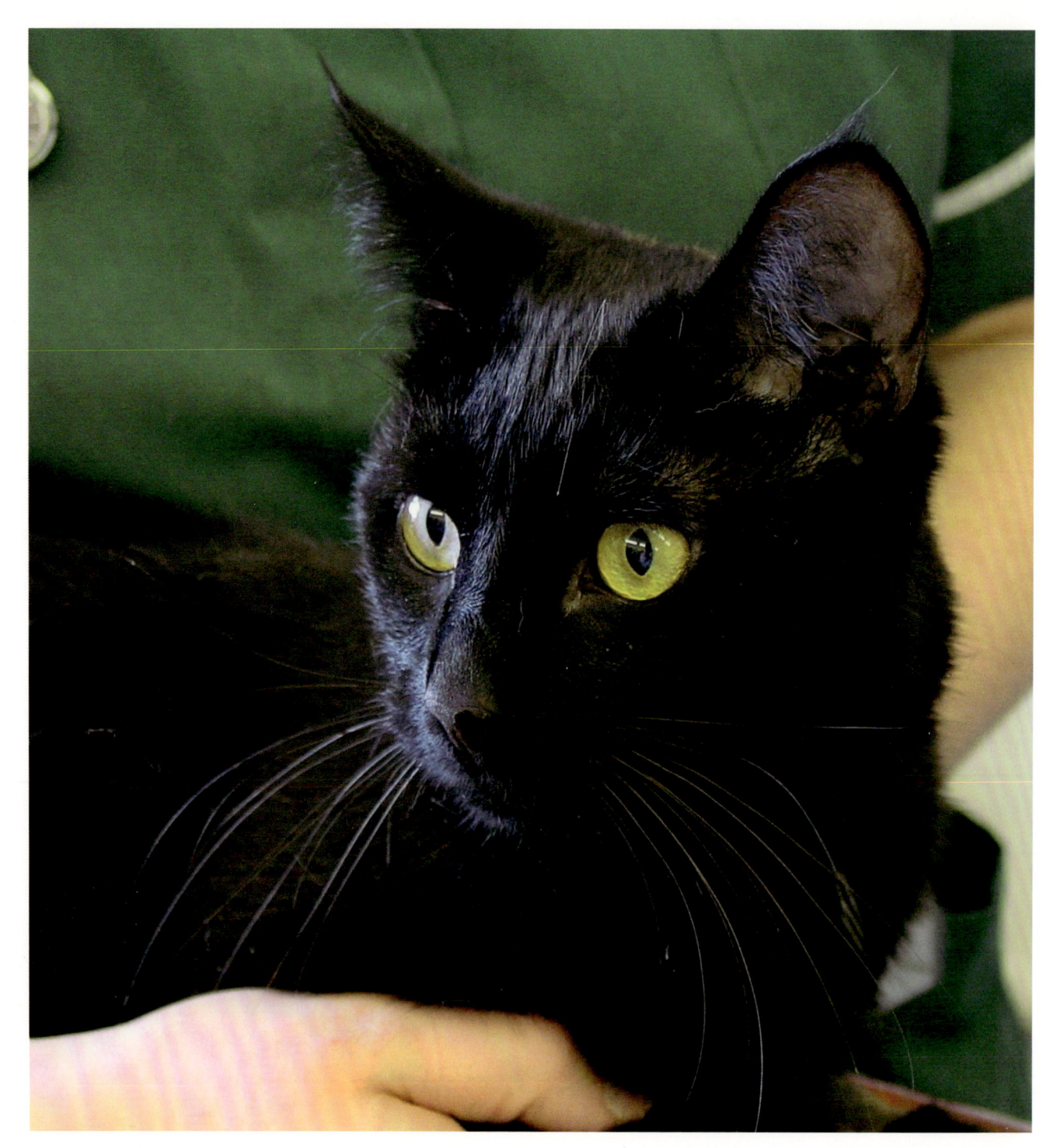